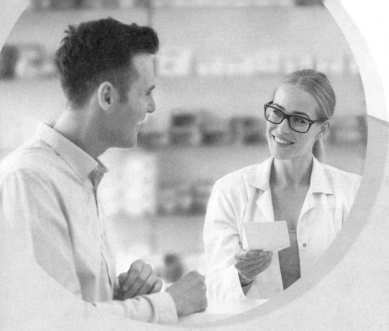

高等学校"十三五"规划教材
新活力英语 高职高专ESP系列

总主编 季舒鸿

药学英语

Pharmaceutical English

主 编 孟 莉
副主编 徐茂红 陈 蕾
编 者 李少兰 刘沛君 李 欣
　　　 梁剑波 周丽丽 徐 睿
　　　 吕长缨 王蕊蕊 吕 斌

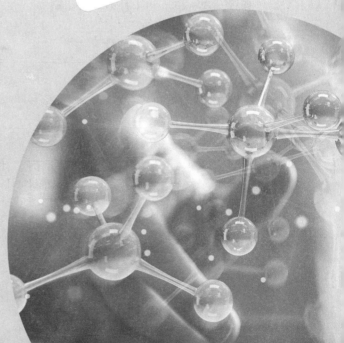

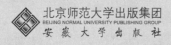

北京师范大学出版集团
安徽大学出版社

图书在版编目(CIP)数据

药学英语/孟莉主编. —合肥:安徽大学出版社,2020.1
(新活力英语. 高职高专 ESP 系列)
ISBN 978-7-5664-1721-3

Ⅰ.①药… Ⅱ.①孟… Ⅲ.①药物学-英语-高等职业教育-教材 Ⅳ.①R9

中国版本图书馆 CIP 数据核字(2019)第 301914 号

药 学 英 语
YAOXUE YINGYU

孟 莉 主编

出版发行:	北京师范大学出版集团 安 徽 大 学 出 版 社 (安徽省合肥市肥西路 3 号 邮编 230039) www.bnupg.com.cn www.ahupress.com.cn
印　　刷:	合肥远东印务有限责任公司
经　　销:	全国新华书店
开　　本:	184 mm×260 mm
印　　张:	8.75
字　　数:	202 千字
版　　次:	2020 年 1 月第 1 版
印　　次:	2020 年 1 月第 1 次印刷
定　　价:	29.80 元

ISBN 978-7-5664-1721-3

策划编辑:葛灵知　　　　　　　　**装帧设计:**李 雪　李 军
责任编辑:葛灵知　韦 玮　李 雪　**美术编辑:**李 军
责任印制:赵明炎

版权所有　侵权必究
反盗版、侵权举报电话:0551—65106311
外埠邮购电话:0551—65107716
本书如有印装质量问题,请与印制管理部联系调换。
印制管理部电话:0551—65106311

Preface
前言

随着经济全球化的发展与跨文化交际的日益增多，国内医药界急需既有专业知识又有较高英语水平的复合型人才。此外，在高等教育体制改革不断深入发展之时，卫生部颁布了《医药卫生中长期人才发展规划(2011-2020)》，这对我国高等药学教育和药学专门人才的培养也提出了更高的要求。近年来，国内药学类专业办学规模不断扩大，办学形式、专业种类和教学方式亦呈多样化发展，高等药学教育进入了新的时期。为适应时代的发展、社会的需求，满足新时期我国高等药学教育的发展要求，加强药学专业英语学习、培养出具备一定跨文化交际能力的复合应用型药学专门人才具有非常重要的意义。药学英语课程正是为实现这一目标而制定的。它是学生在完成公共英语学习之后的延续，旨在培养和提高药学相关专业学生跨文化交际能力的同时，拓展其专业知识面，为日后职业能力的进一步提升打下良好的基础。

遵循高职高专人才培养"实用为主、够用为度"的基本原则，同时结合高等职业院校药学专业学生的就业方向(医疗卫生事业单位、医药制造企业等)，我们组织编写了这本专业信息丰富、实用性强、内容多样化且兼顾专业和英语学习的药学英语教材。

本教材特色体现在：

1. 教材以药学专业知识背景为主线，以提升学生职业能力和职业岗位实践性语言的运用能力为目标；

2. 教材依据高职高专学生总体的英语认知水平进行编排，形式有趣活泼，难度由浅入深、循序渐进，既注重药学专业知识的传授，又重视英语语言能力的提高；

3. 根据药学类相关专业（药学、药物分析、药物制剂、药品经营与管理、中药学等）来设计教材的知识模块，模块下设听说读写和语法内容。选材新颖独特，贴合实际，专业性强但又不失趣味性；

4. 教材一改以往同类教材偏重阅读翻译的惯例，通过真实语言材料将职业情境下的听说练习纳入了学习范畴，并在每个单元设计了专业相关的应用文写作部分，具有广泛的应用性和较高的实用价值；

5. 教材配有同步音频资料，只需扫封面二维码即可获取，随扫随听，便于学习。

本教材可作为高职高专医学类院校药学英语教材，也可供各类医药工作者在职培训或自学使用。

由于编者水平有限，难免存在疏漏和不妥之处，敬请专家和同行批评指正，同时也欢迎使用本教材的广大师生、同仁及医药工作者提出宝贵意见！

编者

2020年1月

★ CONTENTS ★

Unit 1 Drug Administration 1
Lead-in 1
Speaking and Listening 2
  Dialogue   Talking About Drug Safety 2
  Start New Dialogue 2
  Stick Up Your Ears 2
Reading and Writing 3
  In-depth Reading   FDA and CFDA 3
  Practical Writing   Imported Drug License (IDL) 9
Grammar 12
Have Some Fun 15

Unit 2 The History of Pharmacy 16
Lead-in 16
Speaking and Listening 17
  Dialogue   Talking About Major 17
  Start New Dialogue 17
  Stick Up Your Ears 17
Reading and Writing 18
  In-depth Reading   The Early History of Pharmacy 18
  Practical Writing   Summary 26
Grammar 28

Have Some Fun 31

Unit 3 Drug Analysis and Testing 32
　　Lead-in 32
　　Speaking and Listening 33
　　　　Dialogue　　At Drug Analysis Lab 33
　　　　Start New Dialogue 33
　　　　Stick Up Your Ears 33
　　Reading and Writing 34
　　　　In-depth Reading　　Pharmaceutical Analysis 34
　　　　Practical Writing　　Memo 42
　　Grammar 44
　　Have Some Fun 47

Unit 4 Herbal Medicine 48
　　Lead-in 48
　　Speaking and Listening 49
　　　　Dialogue　　Good Medicine Tastes Bitter 49
　　　　Start New Dialogue 49
　　　　Stick Up Your Ears 49
　　Reading and Writing 50
　　　　In-depth Reading　　Herbal Medicine 50
　　　　Practical Writing　　Bar Chart 56
　　Grammar 58
　　Have Some Fun 61

Unit 5 Drug Label 62
　　Lead-in 62
　　Speaking and Listening 63

Dialogue	At the Pharmacy (1)	63
Start New Dialogue		63
Stick Up Your Ears		64

Reading and Writing 64

In-depth Reading	Always Read the Label	64
Practical Writing	A Prescription	71

Grammar 74

Have Some Fun 77

Unit 6 Drug Safety 78

Lead-in 78

Speaking and Listening 79

Dialogue	At the Pharmacy (2)	79
Start New Dialogue		79
Stick Up Your Ears		79

Reading and Writing 80

In-depth Reading	Drug Safety	80
Practical Writing	GMP Certificate	86

Grammar 88

Have Some Fun 91

Unit 7 Drug Development 92

Lead-in 92

Speaking and Listening 93

Dialogue	At the Pharmacy (3)	93
Start New Dialogue		93
Stick Up Your Ears		93

Reading and Writing 94

In-depth Reading	The Drug Development Process	94

Practical Writing　　IND Application Form 100
　　Grammar 102
　　Have Some Fun 105

Unit 8 Pharmaceutical Sales and Marketing 106
　　Lead-in 106
　　Speaking and Listening 107
　　　Dialogue　　Selling a Drug 107
　　　Start New Dialogue 107
　　　Stick Up Your Ears 107
　　Reading and Writing 108
　　　In-depth Reading　　Pfizer: One of the World's Largest Pharmaceutical Companies 108
　　　Practical Writing　　E-mails 114
　　Grammar 116
　　Have Some Fun 120

Glossary 121

References 129

Unit 1 Drug Administration

Lead-in

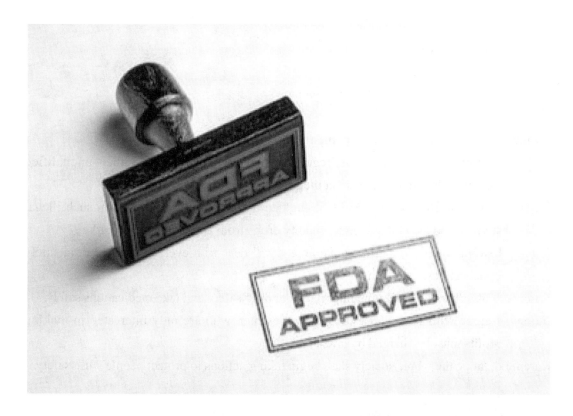

Have you ever known anything about Food and Drug Administration (FDA or US FDA)? FDA affects nearly every American's daily life. It is responsible for protecting the public health by ensuring the safety and efficacy of drugs, medical devices and biological products, as well as the safety of cosmetics and the country's food supply. FDA also has responsibility for enforcing the Federal Food, Drug and Cosmetic Act and several other public health laws.

Speaking and Listening

Dialogue

Talking About Drug Safety

Johnny: Hi, Karen. Recent years, I have heard too much news concerning the quality and safety of drugs in our country, haven't you?

Karen: Oh, yes. The dangerous components cover some drugs we take.

Johnny: There are indeed some companies neglect our country's laws, regulations and standards, having their unqualified products flow into markets via illegal channels.

Karen: I think our government should strengthen its efforts to crack down on such illegal activities and prevent any under-quality drugs from appearing in the market.

Johnny: I strongly believe that the government will deal with every confirmed drug safety cases in a responsible manner.

Karen: All of us should realize the importance of drug safety and take medications safely.

Johnny: I agree with you. Those illegal businessmen who are only interested in making profits must be charged by law.

Karen: I do hope the whole society shall begin taking actions to protect people's life safety.

Start New Dialogue

★ **Discuss and role-play a conversation with your partner based on the given information.**

Imagine you are a senior medical advisor. Start a new dialogue to talk about how the government supervises marketing and selling of medicines in China.

Stick Up Your Ears

★ **Listen to the recording and fill in the blanks according to what you hear.**

The Food and Drug Administration has about nine thousand employees. They

Unit 1 Drug Administration

(1)_____ the manufacture, import, transport, storage and sale of about one million-million dollars worth of products each year. This amount (2)_____ one-fourth of all money spent by American citizens each year.

The agency makes rules for almost ninety-five thousand businesses in the United States. FDA investigators (3)_____ more than fifteen thousand manufacturing centers and farms each year. The investigators make sure that products are made correctly and labeled truthfully. Often, they will collect products for label inspections or (4)_____ by FDA scientists.

The FDA has several choices if a company is found violating any of the laws the agency enforces. FDA officials can urge the company to (5)_____ the problem. Or, they can legally remove, or recall, a bad product from the marketplace. About three thousand products are recalled in the United States each year.

In (6)_____, FDA investigators will seize products if they appear to be unfit for public use. About thirty thousand (7)_____ of imported goods are seized at American ports every year.

The federal government has not always been (8)_____ for the quality of food and drugs in the United States. In the nineteenth century, American states were generally responsible for the safety of locally-made foods and drugs.

Then, Americans began pressuring federal officials to protect resources and set safety (9)_____ for the nation. The Bureau of Chemistry was made responsible for the food and drug (10)_____. The chief chemist at the Bureau was Harvey Wiley. For more than twenty years, he called for a federal law to protect the public from unsafe foods.

Reading and Writing

In-depth Reading

FDA and CFDA

FDA is responsible for protecting the public health by assuring the safety, efficacy and security of human and veterinary drugs, biological products, medical devices, the nation's food supply, cosmetics, and products that emit radiation.

FDA is also responsible for advancing the public health by helping to speed innovations that make medicines more effective, safer, and more affordable and by helping the public get the accurate, science-based information they need to use medicines and foods to maintain and improve their health. FDA also has responsibility for regulating the manufacturing, marketing and distribution of tobacco products to protect the public health and to reduce tobacco use by minors.

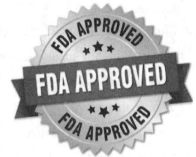

Finally, FDA plays a significant role in the nation's counter terrorism capability. FDA fulfills this responsibility by ensuring the security of the food supply and by fostering development of medical products to respond to deliberate and naturally emerging public health.

The State Food and Drug Administration (SFDA), operates directly under the State Council, China's highest governing body. It is charged with the gigantic task of ensuring the safety of not only foods and drugs, but also the safety of health products and cosmetics. SFDA is charged with exercising administrative and technical supervision over the research, production, marketing and use of whatever is medical—traditional Chinese medicinal materials, prepared herbal drugs, chemical drugs and their raw materials biochemical drugs, bio-products, diagnosis agents, radioactive drugs, anesthetics, toxic drugs, psychotropic substances, medical apparatus, hygiene products and packaging materials for drugs. It is also charged with organizing and coordinating investigations into major accidents caused by unsafe foods, drugs and other products under its jurisdiction.

The China Food and Drug Administration (CFDA) was founded on the basis of the former State Food and Drug Administration (SFDA). In March 2013, the regulatory body was re-branded and restructured as the China Food and Drug Administration, elevating it to a ministerial-level agency. The CFDA replaced a large group of overlapping regulators with an entity similar to the Food and Drug Administration of the United States, streamlining regulation processes for food and drug safety. In March 2018, China's National People's Congress approved plans for the CFDA to be merged into a newly formed National Market Supervision Administration (SAMR). The changes mean that after five years of directly reporting to China's State Council, CFDA will no longer be a stand-alone agency. The agency will cease to exist, with a new National Medical Products Administration (NMPA) being established for regulating drugs and medical devices, under the supervision of the SMRA.

(420 words)

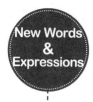

New Words & Expressions

responsible /rɪˈspɒnsəbl/	*adj.*	负有责任的；尽责的；懂道理的
public /ˈpʌblɪk/	*adj.*	公众的，公共的；政府的
	n.	大众；公共场所
safety /ˈseɪftɪ/	*n.*	安全；安全性；安全处所
biological /ˌbaɪəˈlɒdʒɪkl/	*adj.*	生物学的；有血亲关系的
	n.	[药] 生物制品，生物制剂
supply /səˈplaɪ/	*n.*	供给物；储备物质；粮食
cosmetic /kɒzˈmetɪk/	*n.*	化妆品；美发油，发蜡；装饰品；美容术
innovation /ˌɪnəˈveɪʃn/	*n.*	创新；改革；新观念；新事物
affordable /əˈfɔːdəbl/	*adj.*	付得起的
accurate /ˈækjərət/	*adj.*	精确的；准确的；正确无误的
maintain /meɪnˈteɪn/	*vt.*	保持；保养；坚持；固执己见
manufacturing /ˌmænjʊˈfæktʃərɪŋ/	*n.*	制造业，工业
distribution /ˌdɪstrɪˈbjuːʃn/	*n.*	财产分配
significant /sɪɡˈnɪfɪkənt/	*adj.*	有意义的；有重大意义的；值得注意的
	n.	有意义的事物；象征，标志
operate /ˈɒpəreɪt/	*vt.*	经营；运转；管理
	vi.	开刀，动手术
charged /tʃɑːdʒd/	*adj.*	充满感情的；紧张的，可能引起激烈反应的
material /məˈtɪərɪəl/	*n.*	素材；材料，原料；布，织物
biochemical /ˌbaɪəʊˈkemɪkl/	*adj.*	生物化学的
anesthetic /ˌænɪsˈθetɪk/	*n.*	（使局部或全身失去知觉的）麻醉剂，麻醉药
investigation /ɪnˌvestɪˈɡeɪʃn/	*n.*	侦查；调查，研究；科学研究；学术研究
jurisdiction /ˌdʒʊərɪsˈdɪkʃn/	*n.*	管辖权；管辖范围；权限；司法权
play a significant role in		在……发挥重要作用

Notes to the Text

1. FDA is responsible for protecting the public health by assuring the safety, efficacy and security of human and veterinary drugs, biological products, medical devices, our nation's food supply, cosmetics, and products that emit radiation.

解析：此句中 is responsible for 源于短语 be responsible for，意为"对……负责"；by 表示方式、方法；that emit radiation 为后置定语。

译文：FDA 有责任保护公众健康，确保人类和兽类用药、生物制品、医疗器械、食品供应、化妆品和辐射产品的安全性和有效性。

2. FDA is also responsible for advancing the public health by helping to speed innovations that make medicines more effective, safer, and more affordable and by helping the public get the accurate, science-based information they need to use medicines and foods to maintain and improve their health.

解析：speed 在此句中用作动词，意为"加速、促进"；that make medicines more effective, safer, and more affordable 为后置定语从句。

译文：FDA 还负责促进公共卫生，帮助加速创新，使药物更有效、更安全、更便宜，并帮助公众获得使用药物和食品的准确、科学的信息，来维持和改善他们的健康。

3. It is charged with the gigantic task of ensuring the safety of not only foods and drugs but also the safety of health products and cosmetics.

解析：is charged with 在句中表示"负责，肩负……的责任"；not only…but also… 表示"不但……而且……"。

译文：FDA 肩负着确保食品和药品安全重大责任，同时还要负责保健品和化妆品的安全。

4. The agency will cease to exist, with a new National Medical Products Administration (NMPA) being established for regulating drugs and medical devices, under the supervision of the SMRA.

解析：being established for… 为现在分词作后置定语，意为"为了……而建立的……"。

Unit 1 Drug Administration

译文：新组建的国家药品监督管理局（NMPA），负责药品、医疗器械的监督管理工作，由国家市场监督管理总局（SMRA）管理，不再保留国家食品药品监督管理总局。

Post-reading Tasks

I. Answer the following questions according to the text.

1. What is FDA?

2. What are the responsibilities of FDA?

3. What role does FDA play in the Nation's counter terrorism?

4. What is the basis of CFDA?

5. Which department is the competent authority of CFDA?

II. Complete the following statements with the words given below. Change the form if necessary.

significant	operate	cosmetic	biochemical	jurisdiction
accurate	affordable	biological	responsible	innovation

6. The government will be _____ to the President alone.

7. Darwin eventually put forward a model of _____ evolution.

8. Samsung focused primarily on its software _____ and interface inputs such as gesture control and smart scroll/ pause.

9. President Obama said he wanted to create a national healthcare plan that's both easy to use and _____.

10. Seemingly inconsequential （无足轻重的，细琐的）details can sometimes contain_____ clues.

11. Your requirement is outside my _____.

12. Broadcast news was _____ and reliable but sometimes dull.

13. Carbohydrates are one of the four major classes of _____ molecules.

14. These materials mainly used in _____, perfume, hygiene and etc.

15. On the day of Frankie's surgery, the surgeon, Dr. Gregory Zolton, told Jean, "You will have to stay with me while I _____."

III. Read the following passage carefully and choose the best answer.

The Food and Drug Administration has recently proposed severe restrictions on the use of antibiotics（抗生素）to promote the health and growth of meat animals. Medications added to feeds kill many microorganisms, but also encourage the appearance of bacterial strains that are resistant to anti-infective drugs. Already, for example, penicillin（青霉素） and the tetrayclines（四环素）are not as effective therapeutically as they once were. The drug resistance is chiefly conferred by tiny circlets of genes, called plasmids（质粒）, that can be exchanged between different strains and even different species of bacteria. Plasmids are also one of the two kinds of vehicles (the other being viruses) that molecular biologists depend on when performing gene transplant experiments. Even present guidelines forbid the laboratory use of plasmids bearing genes for resistance to antibiotics.

Yet, while congressional debate rages over whether or not to toughen these restrictions on scientists in their laboratories, little congressional attention has been focused on an ill-advised agricultural practice that produces known deleterious effects.

16. In the passage, the author is primarily concerned with _____.

   A. discovering methods of eliminating harmful microorganisms without subsequently generating drug-resistant bacteria

   B. explaining reasons for congressional inaction on the regulation of gene transplant experiments

   C. describing a problematic agricultural practice and its serious genetic consequences

   D. verifying the therapeutic ineffectiveness of anti-infective drugs

17. According to the passage, the exchange of plasmids between different bacteria

can result in which of the following?

   A. Microorganisms resistant to drugs.

   B. Therapeutically useful circlets of genes.

   C. Anti-infective drugs like penicillin.

   D. Viruses for use by molecular biologists.

18. It can be inferred that the author believes that those in favor of stiffening the restrictions on gene transplant research should logically also _____.

    A. encourage experiments with any plasmids except those bearing genes for antibiotic resistance

    B. question the addition of anti-infective drugs to livestock feeds

    C. resist the use of penicillin and tetracyclines to kill microorganisms

    D. agree to the development of meatier live-stock through the use of antibiotics

19. The author's attitude toward the development of bacterial strains that render antibiotic drugs ineffective can best be described as _____.

    A. indifferent

    B. perplexed

    C. pretentious

    D. apprehensive

Practical Writing

Imported Drug License (IDL)

Read and Understand

> The People's Republic of China
>
> **Imported Drug License**
>
> License No. HS********
>
> In accordance with **The Drug Administration Law of P. R. of China** and **The Provisions for Drug Registration**, the following drug produced by the following company has been approved and registered. The importation has been authorized

thereby.

Company: D.H. PHARM. Co., Ltd.　　Country: UK

Address: No.87 Upper Cross Road, London, UK

Generic Name: Compound Vitamin U Tablets　Trade Name: WEISENSU-U

Active Ingredients: Methylmethionine Sulfonium Chloride 25mg, Dried Aluminum Hydroxide Gel 192mg, Magnesium Hydroxide 159mg, Biodiastase 2000 25mg, each tablet.

Dosage Form: Tablets

Strength: Methylmethionine Sulfonium Chloride　25mg/tab

Package Size: 30 tablets / each bottle　Shelf Life: 48 months

Manufacturer: D. H. PHARM. Co., Ltd.

Address: No.87 Upper Cross Road, C　Country: UK

Remarks: 1. Valid Until: Dec. 1, 2023

　　　　　2. Specifications: JX********

China Food and Drug Administration

Dec. 2, 2018

No. 3******

Useful Information

进口药品注册证(Imported Drug License)是经国务院药品监督管理部门组织审查，以确认符合质量标准且安全有效，从而批准进口，并向进口药品的所有人核发注册证书。《进口药品注册证》证号的格式为：H(Z、S) +4位年号 +4位顺序号，其中H代表化学药品，Z代表中药，S代表生物制品。对于境内分包装用大包装规格的注册证，其证号在原注册证号前加字母B。

Generic Name 药品名称	Trade Name 商品名
Active Ingredients 主要成分	Dosage Form 剂型
Strength 规格	Package Size 包装规格
Shelf Life 药品有效期	Remarks 备注

Unit 1 Drug Administration

Writing Practice

Fill the following blanks with the given information.

Flupentixol and Melitracen, which is also known as Deanxit, contain flupentixol (0.5mg) and melitracen (10mg) in each coated tablet. There are 20 tablets in each bottle. The shelf life of the drug is 36 months. The drug is produced by H. Lundbeck A/S, headquartered in Copenhagen, Denmark.

The People's Republic of China

Imported Drug License

License No. HS********

In accordance with The Drug Administration Law of P. R. of China and The Provisions for Drug Registration, the following drug produced by the following company has been approved and registered. The importation has been authorized thereby.

Company: _____

Address: <u>Ottiliavej 9, DK-2500, Valby, Denmark</u>   Country: _____

Generic Name: _____ Trade Name: _____

Active Ingredients: _____

Dosage Form: _____ Strength: _____

Package Size: _____ Shelf Life: _____

Manufacturer: _____

Address: <u>Ottiliavej 9, DK-2500, Valby, Denmark</u>   Country: _____

Remarks: 1. Valid Until: _____

     2. Specifications: JX********

China Food and Drug Administration

Dec. 2, 2019

No. 3******

Grammar

Attributive Clause
定语从句

在现代汉语里定语一般都放在中心词的前面，但是在英语里为了句子的平衡，常常把定语放在所修饰词之后，这种情况叫做定语后置，这样的定语叫做后置定语。后置定语可以分为五大类：1. 定语从句作后置定语；2. 非谓语动词作后置定语；3. 介词短语作后置定语；4. 形容词短语作后置定语；5. 单个词作后置定语。我们先来介绍第一类定语从句作后置定语。

在复合句中，修饰某一名词或代词的从句叫定语从句。被修饰的名词或代词叫先行词（antecedent），定语从句一般放在先行词的后面。

定语从句一般由关系代词或关系副词来引导，关系词放在先行词与定语从句之间起连接作用，同时又作从句中的某个成分。

1. 关系代/副词

引导定语从句的关联词包括关系代词和关系副词。

关系代词（relative pronoun）：that，which，who，whom，whose；

关系副词（relative adverb）：when，where，why。

关系代词	指代	从句中成分	例句
that	人或物	主语或宾语	The train which/that has just left is for Shenzhen.
who	人	主语或宾语	He is the man who lives next door.
whom	人	宾语	The man whom we have just seen is a writer.
whose	人或物	定语	He is the man whose car was stolen last week.
which	物	主语或宾语	That was the clue which clinched it for us.

关系副词	指代	例句
when	时间	I still remember the time when we first met.
where	地点	This is the hotel where they are staying.
why	原因	That is the reason why he is leaving so soon.

2. 限制性定语从句和非限制性定语从句

（1）限制性定语从句（restrictive attributive clause）说明先行词的情况，对先行词起限定作用，与先行词关系十分密切，不可用逗号隔开，也不可省略，否则全句意义就不完整。

This is the telegram which he refers to.

这就是他提到的电报。

（2）非限制性定语从句（non-restrictive attributive clause）只是对先行词作补充说明，没有限定作用，通常用逗号与主句隔开。它与先行词的关系比较松散，若省略，原句的意义依然完整。引导非限制性定语从句的关系词有：who, whom, whose, which, when 和 where，不可以用 that 和 why。

The book was left by Tom, who was here a moment ago.

这本书是汤姆的，刚才他还在这儿。

As a boy, he was always making things, most of which were electric.

作为男孩，他喜欢做东西，做的大多数都是电子的。

（3）两种定语从句的内涵不同，限制性定语从句具有涉他性，而非限制性定语从句具有唯一性，这在理解和翻译时应特别注意。试比较：

His brother, who is eighteen years old, is a PLA man.

他的哥哥是个解放军战士，现年十八岁。（说明他只有一个哥哥）

His brother who is a PLA man is eighteen years old.

他那个十八岁的哥哥是个解放军。（说明他还有别的哥哥）

Exercises

I. Fill in the blanks with the correct relative pronouns.

1. The man _____ wallet was stolen is very upset.

2. The book _____ was lying on the table is mine.

3. Is there a shop near here _____ sells cigarette?

4. I'm afraid that's all _____ I can do for you.

5. My sister, you spoke to _____ at the party, wants to study history.

II. Choose the best answer for each of the following sentences.

6. Do you know the man _____?

   A. whom I spoke

   B. to who spoke

   C. I spoke to

   D. that I spoke

7. That is the day _____ I'll never forget.

   A. which

   B. on which

   C. in which

   D. when

8. This is the hotel last month _____.

   A. which they stayed

   B. at that they stayed

   C. where they stayed at

   D. where they stayed

9. This is one of the best films _____.

   A. that have been shown this year

   B. that have shown

   C. that has been shown this year

   D. that you talked

10. The pen _____ he is writing is mine.

    A. with which

    B. in which

    C. on which

    D. by which

III. Translate a passage from Chinese into English and try to use attributive clauses.

FDA 是食品药品监督管理局（Food and Drug Administration）的简称。FDA 有时也代表美国 FDA，即美国食品药品监督管理局。美国 FDA 是国际医疗审核权威机构，由美国国会即联邦政府授权，专门从事食品与药品管理的最高执法机关；是一个由医生、律师、微生物学家、药理学家、化学家和统计学家等专业人士组成的致力于保护、促进和提高国民健康的政府卫生管制的监控机构。其他许多国家都通过寻求和接收 FDA 的帮助来促进并监控其本国产品的安全。

参考词汇：

权威机构 authority；执法机关 law enforcement agency；

监控机构 monitoring institution

Have Some Fun

A pharmacist goes to a nursing home to review an elderly customer. As he is sitting there, he notices a bowl of peanuts beside her bed and takes one. As they talk, he can't help himself and eats one after another. By the time they are through talking, the bowl is empty.

He says, "Ma'am, I'm sorry, but I seem to have eaten all of your peanuts."

"That's okay," she says. "They would have just sat there. Without my teeth, all I can do is to suck the chocolate off and put them back."

Unit 2 The History of Pharmacy

Lead-in

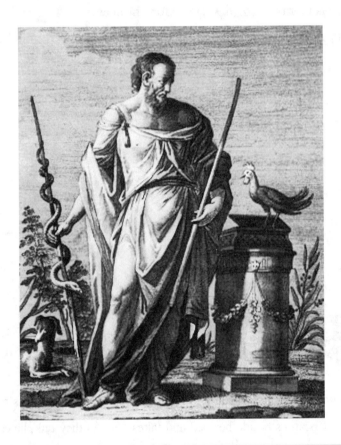

Pharmacy is the science and technique of preparing and dispensing drugs. It is a health profession that links health sciences with chemical sciences and aims to ensure the safe and effective use of pharmaceutical drugs. Have you ever known anything about the history of pharmacy? Do you know anyone who contributed to the development of pharmacy? You can find out answers to the questions in this unit.

Unit 2 The History of Pharmacy

Speaking and Listening

Dialogue

Talking About Major

Sara: Hi, Linda!

Linda: Hi, Sara. Nice to meet you again.

Sara: I hope you are settling in (适应) at college!

Linda: I am! I've made a lot of friends and I really enjoy my courses.

Sara: Good! Me too! By the way, what are you studying here?

Linda: I'm studying Pharmacy here.

Sara: Really? That's great! Do you hope to join a company manufacturing drugs after graduating?

Linda: Maybe. My parents run a pharmacy in my hometown. They hope I can help them run it after graduation. But I want to get a job in Shanghai. It's too soon to say really. What about you?

Sara: I'm studying nursing here. I dream to be a good nurse.

Start New Dialogue

★ Discuss and role-play a conversation with your partner based on the given information.

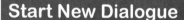

You are a freshman at college. You and your classmate are talking about your major (pharmacy/pharmaceutical analysis/Chinese pharmacological specialty/medicinal marketing, etc).

Stick Up Your Ears

★ Listen to the recording and fill in the blanks according to what you hear.

Careers in pharmacy offer many benefits and opportunities. These include

17

(1)_____ in the community, a hospital, home health care, pharmaceutical research companies, nursing homes, government health agencies, and higher education. Pharmacists play (药师) a (2)_____ role in improving patient care through the medicine and information they provide. Pharmacy is a well-rounded career blending science, (3)_____, direct patient contact, computer technology and business. In addition, pharmacy has (4)_____ earning potential and is consistently ranked as one of the most highly trusted professions due to the care and service pharmacists provide. A PharmD (药学博士) degree can be (5)_____ to diverse careers. Clinical pharmacists promote appropriate, effective and safe medication use for patients. By working as part of a health care team, pharmacists are able to closely (6)_____ patient drug therapy and make recommendations on the selection of the best medication (用药) for a patient's condition, the correct dose (剂量), and the duration of therapy.

Some community pharmacists provide (7)_____ services to help patients manage conditions such as diabetes (糖尿病), asthma (哮喘), smoking cessation (戒烟), or high blood pressure. Community pharmacists are the most (8)_____ branch of practice advising patients on the proper use of their prescription and non-prescription medication use, and keeping records of their patient's health, illnesses, and medications. A hospital pharmacist advises other health professionals about the actions, interactions, and (9)_____ of drugs, and counsels patients about medications. They advise physicians and other health practitioners (医师) on the selection, (10)_____, interactions, and side effects of medications.

Reading and Writing

In-depth Reading

The Early History of Pharmacy

Before the Dawn of History

Ancient man learned from instinct, from observation of birds and beasts. Cool water, a leaf, dirt, or mud was his first soothing application. By trial, he learned which served him best. Eventually, he applied his knowledge for the benefit of others. Despite the crude methods, many of today's medicines spring from sources which were within reach of early man.

Egyptian Medicine (2900 B.C.)

Though Egyptian medicine dates from about 2900 B.C., best known and most important pharmaceutical record is the "Papyrus Ebers" (1500 B.C.), a collection of 800 prescriptions, mentioning 700 drugs. Pharmacy in ancient Egypt was conducted by gatherers and preparers of drugs, and head pharmacists. They are thought to have worked in the "House of Life".

Pharmacy in Ancient Babylonia (2600 B.C.)

Babylonia and Ninoi were two cities that cradled such civilization. Medical texts recorded first the symptoms of illness, the prescription and directions for compounding, then an invocation to the gods. Ancient Babylonian methods find counterpart in today's modern pharmaceutical, medical, and spiritual care of the sick.

Pharmacy in Ancient China (2000 B.C.)

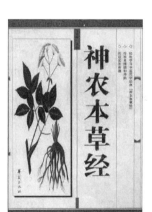

Chinese Pharmacy, according to legend, stems from Shen Nong (about 2000 B.C.), emperor who sought out and investigated the medicinal value of several hundred herbs. He is reputed to have tested many of them on himself, and to have laid foundation for the first *Pen T-Sao*, or *Native Herbs*, recording 365 drugs.

Theophrastus — Father of Botany (300 B.C.)

Theophrastus (about 300 B.C.), among the greatest early Greek philosophers and natural scientists, is called the "Father of Botany". His observations and writings dealing with the medical qualities and peculiarities of herbs are unusually accurate, even in the light of present knowledge. His most famous book is *Plant Explanations*.

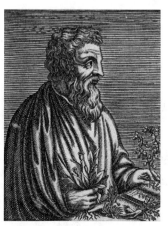

Dioscorides — a Scientist Looks at Drugs (100 A.D.)

Pedanios Dioscorides, a Greek physician, (first century A.D.), contributed mightily to the transition in from the level of vocation to science pharmacy. In order to study materia medica, Dioscorides accompanied the Roman armies throughout the known world. He recorded what he observed, promulgated excellent rules for collection of drugs, their storage and use. In his book, *Materia Medica*, he described about 600 herbs and some drugs. His texts were considered basic science as late as the sixteenth century.

Galen — Experimenter in Drug Compounding

Of the men of ancient times whose names were known and revered among both the professions of pharmacy and medicine, Galen, undoubtedly, was the foremost. Galen (130~200 A.D.) is a Greek scientist born in Pergamon in minor Asia. Galen's principles of preparing and compounding medicines ruled in the western world for 1,500 years; and his name still is associated with compounded pharmaceuticals—galenicals. He was the originator of the formula for a cold cream, essentially similar to that known today. Many procedures Galen originated have their counterparts in today's modern compounding laboratories.

(485 words)

New Words & Expressions

pharmacy /ˈfɑːməsɪ/	n.	药房；配药学，药剂学
instinct /ˈɪnstɪŋkt/	n.	本能，直觉；天性
/ɪnˈstɪŋkt/	adj.	充满着的
application /ˌæplɪˈkeɪʃn/	n.	申请（表，书）；应用
eventually /ɪˈventʃʊəlɪ/	adv.	终于，最后
Egyptian /ɪˈdʒɪpʃn/	n.	埃及人
	adj.	埃及的
invocation /ˌɪnvəˈkeɪʃn/	n.	祈求，祈祷
promulgate /ˈprɒmlɡeɪt/	vt.	公布；传播；发表
revere /rɪˈvɪə(r)/	v.	崇敬，尊敬
galenical /ɡəˈlenɪkəl/	n.	草药，未经精炼的药物
	adj.	草本制剂的
spring from		起源于，来自，发源（于）……
be thought to		被认为
stem from		起源于
in the light of		根据，按照

Unit 2 The History of Pharmacy

contribute to	有助于；贡献
as late as	迟至……才，一直到
be associated with	与……有关，涉及
Theophrastus	泰奥弗拉斯托斯（古希腊哲学家、自然科学家）
Shen Nong	神农（又称神农氏，神话人物，远古传说中的太阳神，被世人尊称为"药王""五谷王""五谷先帝""神农大帝""地皇"等）
Pen T-Sao	《神农本草经》（我国第一部药学专著，大约成书于秦汉时期，全书共分三卷，载药365种，其中植物药252种，动物药67种，矿物药46种）
Father of Botany	植物学之父
Pedanios Dioscorides	迪奥斯科里德（公元1世纪时罗马军队的外科医生）
Materia Medica	《药物论》（公元1世纪希腊医生迪奥斯克里德斯的著作，是欧洲1600年间的药物学基础）
Pergamon	帕加马（古国名，位于小亚细亚西北）

Notes to the Text

1. Despite their crude methods, many of today's medicines spring from sources which were within reach of early man.

解析：despite 为介词，此处构成介词短语位于句首，此句意为"尽管他们的方法很原始"；主句中 which 引导的从句为 those 的后置定语。

译文：尽管他们（发现药物）的方法很原始，但如今很多药物都来源于古人的发现。

2. Though Egyptian medicine dates from about 2900 B.C., best known and most important pharmaceutical record is the "Papyrus Ebers" (1500 B.C.), a collection of 800 prescriptions, mentioning 700 drugs.

解析：a collection of 800 prescriptions, mentioning 700 drugs 是 Papyrus Ebers 的同位语，其中 mentioning 700 drugs 相当于非限制性定语从句 which mentions 700 drugs。

译文：虽然埃及的药物史可追溯到公元前2900年，但最广为人知，也是最重要的药典则是公元前1500年出现的《爱柏氏纸草纪事》。书中记录了800种处方，涉及700种药物。

3. He is reputed to have tested many of them on himself, and to have laid foundation for the first *Pen T-Sao*, or *Native Herbs*, recording 365 drugs.

解析：词组 be reputed to have done sth. 意为"普遍认为，号称"；to have laid foundation 为固定短语，意为"打下基础"；recording 365 drugs 同样为动词现在分词引导的后置定语从句，相当于 which records。

译文：他以亲身尝试许多种草药而闻名于世，并且为撰写第一本药书《神农本草经》（又名《本草经》）打下基础。这本药书记录了365种药物。

4. His observations and writings dealing with the medical qualities and peculiarities of herbs are unusually accurate, even in the light of present knowledge.

解析：dealing with the medical qualities and peculiarities of herbs 为现在分词作后置定语，相当于 which deal with…；in the light of 介词短语，意为"根据、鉴于"。

译文：即便是依据人类现有的认知，他对于草药品质特性的观察与记录都是极为准确的。

5. Of the men of ancient times whose names are known and revered among both the professions of Pharmacy and Medicine, Galen, undoubtedly, is the foremost.

解析：of the men… 意为"在……人中"；whose 在句中引导后置定语从句。

译文：毫无疑问，在药学和医学界备受尊重的古代名人中，伽林是最杰出的。

Unit 2 The History of Pharmacy

Post-reading Tasks

I. Answer the following questions according to the text.

1. How did ancient people discover medicines from nature?
   _____

2. What do medical texts first record in ancient Babylonia?
   _____

3. What did Shen Nong contribute to Chinese pharmacy?
   _____

4. How did Pedanios Dioscorides study materia medica?
   _____

II. Complete the following statements with the words or phrases given below. Change the form if necessary.

| worship | instinct | stem from | eventually | contribute to |
| associate | peculiarity | essentially | promulgate | create |

5. God reminds his people that He is to be _____.

6. He seems so honest and genuine and my every _____ says he's not.

7. Confidence and fear are contradictory states of mind that both _____ our belief and attitudes.

8. It was a hard journey but his ship _____ reached a continent.

9. These efforts _____ our understanding of the virus, its patterns of spread, and the spectrum of sickness it can cause.

10. Sowing the seeds of tomorrow so that future generations can _____ a more sustainable world.

11. It makes sense that daytime sleepiness would be _____ with depression.

12. It is the _____ of knowledge that those who really thirst for it always get it.

13. The Comfort is, _____, a floating hospital.

14. A new constitution was _____ last month.

III. Read the following passage carefully and choose the best answer.

Clinical pharmacists work directly with physicians, other health professionals, and patients to ensure that the medications prescribed for patients contribute to the best possible health outcomes. Clinical pharmacists practice in health care settings where they have frequent and regular interactions with physicians and other health professionals, contributing to better coordination of care.

The clinical pharmacist is educated and trained in direct patient care environments, including medical centers, clinics, and a variety of other health care settings. Clinical pharmacists are frequently granted patient care privileges by collaborating physicians and/or health systems that allow them to perform a full range of medication decision-making functions as part of the patient's health care team. These privileges are granted on the basis of the clinical pharmacist's demonstrated knowledge of medication therapy and record of clinical experience. This specialized knowledge and clinical experience is usually gained through residency training and specialist board certification. Clinical pharmacists are required to:

* Assess the status of the patient's health problems and determine whether the prescribed medications are optimally meeting the patient's needs and goals of care.
* Evaluate the appropriateness and effectiveness of the patient's medications.
* Recognize untreated health problems that could be improved or resolved with appropriate medication therapy.
* Follow the patient's progress to determine the effects of the patient's medications on his or her health.
* Consult with the patient's physicians and other health care providers in selecting the medication therapy that best meets the patient's needs and contributes effectively to the overall therapy goals.
* Advise the patient on how to best take his or her medications.
* Support the health care team's efforts to educate the patient on other important steps to improve or maintain health, such as exercise, diet, and preventive steps like immunization.

* Refer the patient to his or her physician or other health professionals to address specific health, wellness, or social services concerns as they arise.

Clinical pharmacists care for patients by:

* Provide a consistent process of patient care that ensures the appropriateness, effectiveness, and safety of the patient's medication use.

* Consult with the patient's physician(s) and other health care provider(s) to develop and implement a medication plan that can meet the overall goals of patient care established by the health care team.

* Apply specialized knowledge of the scientific and clinical use of medications, including medication action, dosing, adverse effects, and drug interactions, in performing their patient care activities in collaboration with other members of the health care team.

* Call on their clinical experience to solve health problems through the rational use of medications.

* Rely on their professional relationships with patients to tailor their advice to best meet individual patient needs and desires.

15. Clinical pharmacists practice in health care settings to _____.

    A. study some courses about pharmacy

    B. have interactions with patients

    C. get more communication with physicians and other health professionals

    D. collect cases for research on drug development

16. Clinical pharmacists are often permitted to _____.

    A. collaborate physicians and/or health systems

    B. prescribe all medications after completing a training program

    C. educated and trained in the health care settings

    D. perform a full range of medication decision-making functions

17. Which of the following statements is NOT true?

    A. Clinical pharmacists select the medication therapy for patients.

    B. Clinical pharmacists suggest the patient on how to best take his or her drugs.

    C. Clinical pharmacists evaluate the condition of the patient's health problems.

D. Clinical pharmacists educate the patient on exercise, diet and preventive steps.

18. The knowledge of the scientific and clinical use of medications used by clinical pharmacists in performing their patient care activities doesn't include _____.

    A. medication action   B. adverse effects

    C. drug interactions   D. indications

Practical Writing

Summary

Read and Understand

Original:

I went to the drugstore down the street to fill a prescription at the pharmacy. I have had some problems with my arm and the doctor prescribed for me a new medication. I waited in line and when it was my turn, I handed the prescription to the pharmacist. She told me to come back in 15 minutes and she would have it ready for me.

In the meantime, I went to look for some over the counter stomach medication. There was some in tablets and capsules. I decided on the capsules and returned to the pharmacy.

The pharmacist asked me if I had taken this medication before. I told her I hadn't, and she pointed out the directions on the bottle. It had the dosage information: Take two tablets two times a day. There was also a warning to not take it on an empty stomach. The bottle also said that I should stop taking the medication if I had any serious side effects. The pharmacist told me to follow the directions closely so that I can avoid an overdose. I paid for the medication and thanked her for her help.

Summary:

I went to a pharmacy to fill a prescription which was prescribed by the doctor to solve some problems with my arm. The pharmacist filled the prescription for me and told me how to take the medicine. Finally, I paid for the medicine and expressed my gratitude to the pharmacist.

Writing Skills

Five Steps to Write a Summary

Step 1: Skim the text to find out the general theme.

Step 2: Analyse the text's structure to divide it into several sections, find out the main idea of each section and write it out briefly with your own words (one sentence).

Step 3: Write down the key supporting points for each main idea without involving minor details.

Step 4: Organize the main and related supporting points in a logical order with necessary transitions to achieve coherence.

Step 5: Proofread for grammatical, spelling and punctuation mistakes.

Writing Practice

Write a Summary of the following passage.

In order to become a pharmacist it requires attending Pharmacy school or college. The way I graduated from Pharmacy school was to go to community college for two years, get an associate's degree in Math and Science and then transfer those credits to Arnold and Marie Schwartz College of Pharmacy. When I went to Pharmacy school it was a six-year course. It's now a seven-year one.

The more traditional way to do it is to graduate out of high school, get accepted to a pharmacy school and do the entire program with your core sciences and the pharmacy program all in one. So, typically, it's two years of pre-pharmacy. And, then, what was four years, now five years of Pharmaceutical studies. So, your Pharmaceutical Chemistry. It's the physiology, the math, and it's now a seven-year program. In your last year of school, you usually do a residency and an internship. So, they want you to work in a hospital setting and in a retail setting. And then, when you finish your rotations, you'll take boards. There's a compounding board, there's a written exam, and there's a law exam. And once you've completed those, they issue your license.

Summary (no more than 70 words):

_____

_____

_____

_____

_____

Grammar

Present Participle Used as Attributive
现在分词作定语

现在分词短语常用作名词的后置定语，与中心名词构成逻辑主谓关系，可以转换为定语从句。

The building **sitting on Alcatraz Island** was a federal prison.

坐落在恶魔岛的那栋房子曾经是一所联邦监狱。

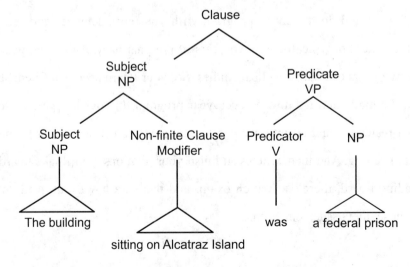

= The building **that sits on Alcatraz Island** was a federal prison.

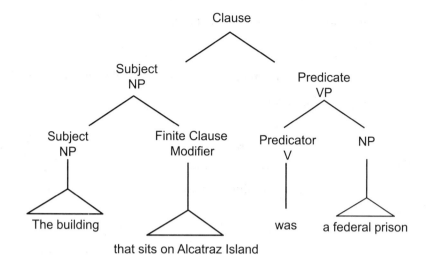

现在分词作后置定语有时表示其逻辑主语动作的正在进行，有时则用以描述逻辑主语客观永恒的状态或性质。

The girl **holding up an umbrella** was afraid the rain might spoil her new hat.

打着伞的那个女孩担心雨会淋坏她的新帽子。

The young man **sitting between John and Mary** is the editor of the campus newspaper.

坐在约翰和玛丽之间的那个年轻小伙子是校报的编辑。

He is reputed to have tested many of them on himself, and to have made great contribution for the first *Pen T-Sao*, or *Native Herbs*, **recording 365 drugs**.

人们认为他亲身尝过很多种草药，并为第一本记录了365种药物的《神农本草经》（又称《本草经》）做出了巨大贡献。

His observations and writings **dealing with the medical qualities and peculiarities of herbs** are unusually accurate, even in the light of present knowledge.

即便是依据现在的知识水平，他那些有关草药医学品质和特性的观察记录仍然十分准确。

Exercises

I. Rewrite the following sentences using present participle phrases.

1. Can you think of the name of a flower which begins with " t "?

2. Those who wish to join the club should sign here.

3. The best known and most important pharmaceutical record is the "Papyrus Ebers" (1500 B.C.), which mentions 700 drugs.

4. The man who was wearing a blue shirt and blue jeans was caught shortly after he had left the bank.

5. The professor who is giving a speech now is from Harvard University.

II. Read the following statements carefully, and tick the ones including present participle phrases used as post-positive attributives.

☐ 6. There are lots of places of interest needing to be repaired in our city.

☐ 7. Walking on the beach is painful if jellyfish have washed ashore.

☐ 8. A few days after the interview, I received a letter offering me the job.

☐ 9. Waking to the buzz of the alarm clock, Freddie cursed the arrival of another Monday.

☐ 10. The subject interesting him at the moment is Greek history.

III. Translate a passage from Chinese into English and try to use at least one present participle phrase as post-positive attributive in your translation.

《本草纲目》是明代著名的医学家李时珍所著。这部著作近 200 万字，记载药物 1892 种。除了中草药，该书也包含了动物和矿物质作为药物的记载。《本草纲目》堪称中医史上最完整的医书，对各种药物的名称、气味、形态等都做了详尽的介绍。它被翻译成 20 多种语言并在全世界广为流传。即使到现在，人们还常常将它用作医学参考书。

参考词汇：

《本草纲目》*Compendium of Materia Medica*；中草药 Chinese herbal medicine

Have Some Fun

Sickness is felt, but health not at all. — T. Fuller
疾病是可以感觉到的，但健康则完全不。—— 富勒
An apple a day keeps the doctor away.
每天一苹果，医生远离我。
Early to bed and early to rise, makes a man healthy, wealthy and wise. — Benjamin Franklin
早睡早起，使人健康、富有、明智。—— 本杰明·富兰克林

Unit 3 Drug Analysis and Testing

Lead-in

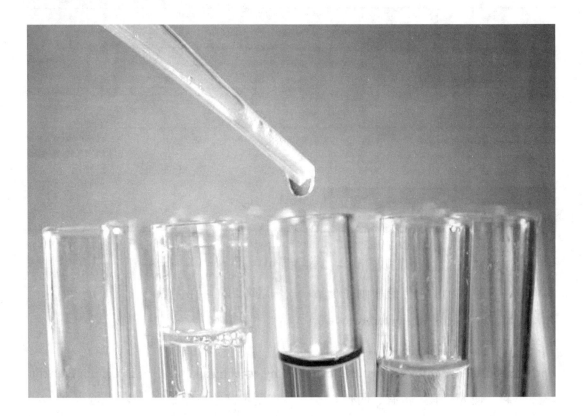

Drug analysis is an important part of analytical chemistry. It focuses on qualitative and quantitative analysis of drugs, quality control as well as development of new drugs by using methods and techniques in physics, chemistry, biology and microbiology. The science is widely applied in a number of fields, including drug quality control, clinical pharmacy and analysis of traditional Chinese medicine and natural drugs, etc. Have you ever known anything about how drug analysis is conducted? And do you know any instrumental methods that can be used to carry out drug analysis?

Speaking and Listening

Dialogue

At Drug Analysis Lab

Jessica: Excuse me, do you know where the drug analysis lab is?

Ellen: Yes. It's just on the fifth floor of this building.

Jessica: How often do you perform drug analysis experiments there?

Ellen: Almost every day, because we need enough practical exercises to know how drug analysis is conducted.

Jessica: Can you go there without a teacher?

Ellen: No. That's not allowed.

Jessica: What does the teacher often tell you to do when you are doing an experiment?

Ellen: He often tells us to follow the instructions and take good care of the instruments.

Jessica: What will you do when you finish the experiment?

Ellen: We are expected to put everything back in the proper place and wash our hands.

Jessica: Right. It is very important to keep the lab clean.

Ellen: Yes, safe as well. We also have to make sure the electricity is cut off and the windows are shut before leaving.

Start New Dialogue

★ Discuss and role-play a conversation with your partner based on the given information.

In a laboratory, you are asking your teacher about what you should pay attention to when you are in the drug analysis lab before conducting an experiment.

Stick Up Your Ears

★ Listen to the recording and fill in the blanks according to what you hear.

Working as a laboratory analyst is often (1) _____ for people who are fascinated by science and enjoy performing scientific experiments. These individuals analyze (2) _____ specimens (样本) and can work in a variety of settings, including hospitals and industrial facilities. Some common job duties of a laboratory analyst include conducting experiments, recording results, cleaning testing equipment, maintaining laboratory safety and monitoring inventory (监测库存).

The (3) _____ responsibility of a laboratory analyst is conducting experiments. For example, if he is working at a hospital, he might perform testing on patients' tissue samples. If he is working at an industrial facility, he may do testing on different chemicals used in production.

Upon the (4) _____ of an experiment or testing, an individual will be required to record the results. In the case of a tissue sample, he might need to (5) _____ if it was cancerous (癌性的) and document his findings. Most of the time, the results will be placed in a database so they can be easily (6) _____ by computer in the future. After each test, a laboratory analyst will also need to (7) _____ any leftover wastes. When appropriate, he might also publish his findings in scientific journals for other (8) _____ to review.

Along with this, it's important for a laboratory analyst to clean testing equipment. Items like beakers, flasks, test tubes and other materials all need to be cleaned to (9) _____ hazards or incorrect test results.

Maintaining laboratory safety is another duty of a laboratory analyst. Due to the use of (10) _____ chemicals and the potential for accidents, he must inspect equipment and keep the lab clean. If he finds faulty equipment or other hazards, it's his job to address the situation and report it to a supervisor.

Reading and Writing

In-depth Reading

Pharmaceutical Analysis

A pharmaceutical analysis is intended to either identify or quantify one or more substances in a given sample. The substance to be identified or quantified is called the analyte. The samples in drug analysis are typically pharmaceutical raw materials, finished pharmaceutical products or biological samples like human blood or urine which contain one or more drug substances. The samples consist of one or several analytes, and a sample matrix which is the rest of the sample. Identification, also referred to as qualitative analysis, is intended to confirm the identity of the analytes. A quantitative analysis, also termed as determination, is intended to measure the exact concentration or the exact amount of the analyte in a given sample.

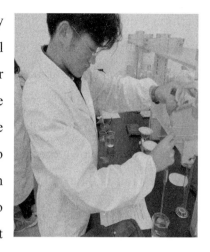

As an example, paracetamol tablets containing 500 mg paracetamol per tablet have to be controlled prior to release from production. This is accomplished by pharmaceutical analysis. Paracetamol is the analyte, whereas the rest of tablet, consisting of different pharmaceutical excipients, is the sample matrix. Identification of paracetamol in the tablets is performed to make sure that the tablets contain the correct active pharmaceutical ingredient, whereas a quantitative analysis is performed to measure the content of paracetamol and to check that this result is exactly or close to 500 mg per tablet. In the latter case, a determination of paracetamol is performed.

There are numerous qualitative chemical tests, for example, the acid test for gold and the Kastle-Meyer test for the presence of blood. Most commonly, and historically, a strong acid is used in the acid test for gold to distinguish gold from base metals. The Kastle-Meyer test for the presence of blood is often used in television crime dramas to show the presence of blood at a crime scene. Evidence that appears to be blood is tested to determine if it is actually blood, and not something that just looks like blood. A flame test, which is an analytic procedure performed in chemistry to detect the presence of certain elements, primarily metal ions, based on each element's particular emission spectrum, is also a type of qualitative analysis.

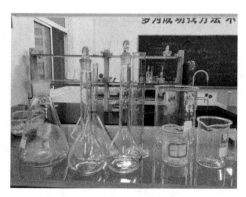

For quantitative analysis, an analyst has to

perform a qualitative analysis prior to performing the more difficult quantitative analysis. It is normally performed in terms of weight and volume. Gravimetric analysis involves determining the amount of material present by weighing the sample before and/or after some transformation. In most cases, a quantitative pharmaceutical analysis is performed when the analyte is present in a solution. Therefore, titration, also known as titrimetry, is used to determine the unknown concentration of an identified analyte. Since volume measurements play a key role in titration, it is also known as volumetric analysis.

(439 words)

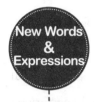

New Words & Expressions

identify /aɪˈdentɪfaɪ/	vt.	鉴定；识别，辨认出；把……看成一样
	vi.	认同；感同身受
substance /ˈsʌbstəns/	n.	物质，材料；实质，内容；（织品的）质地
sample /ˈsɑːmpl/	n.	样品；标本；榜样
	vt.	取……的样品，抽样调查
analyte /ænəˈlaɪt/	n.	（被）分析物；分解物
raw /rɔː/	adj.	生的，未加工的；无经验的
matrix /ˈmeɪtrɪks/	n.	[数]矩阵；模型
quantitative /ˈkwɒntɪtətɪv/	adj.	定量的；数量（上）的
amount /əˈmaʊnt/	n.	量，数量；总额
	vi.	等于；等同，接近；合计，总共
paracetamol /ˌpærəˈsiːtəmɒl/	n.	对乙酰氨基酚；氨基酚
tablet /ˈtæblət/	n.	碑，匾；药片；便笺簿；小块
release /rɪˈliːs/	vt.	释放，放开；发布，发行
	n.	释放，排放，解除
excipient /ɪkˈsɪpiənt/	n.	赋型剂；药用辅料
ingredient /ɪnˈɡriːdiənt/	n.	（混合物的）组成部分；要素；因素；（烹调的）原料

Unit 3 Drug Analysis and Testing

numerous /ˈnjuːmərəs/	adj.	很多的，许多的；数不清的
determine /dɪˈtɜːmɪn/	v.	决定；确定；测定
procedure /prəˈsiːdʒə(r)/	n.	程序，手续；工序，步骤
detect /dɪˈtekt/	vt.	查明，发现；侦查
element /ˈelɪmənt/	n.	要素；元素；（学科的）基本原则
primarily /praɪˈmerəlɪ/	adv.	首先；首要地，主要地；根本上
particular /pəˈtɪkjələ(r)/	adj.	特定的；专指的；特殊的；特别的；挑剔的
emission /ɪˈmɪʃn/	n.	排放，辐射；排放物，散发物（尤指气体）
spectrum /ˈspektrəm/	n.	光谱，波谱；范围；系列
gravimetric /ˌɡrævɪˈmetrɪk/	adj.	（测定）重量的，重量分析的
transformation /ˌtrænsfəˈmeɪʃn/	n.	转化；转变；改造；转型
solution /səˈluːʃn/	n.	解决；溶解，溶液；答案
titration /taɪˈtreɪʃn/	n.	滴定；滴定法；滴定法测定
titrimetry /taɪˈtrɪmɪtrɪ/	n.	滴定分析；滴定测量，滴定分析法
consist of		由……组成；包括
prior to		在……之前
distinguish from		辨别；将……与……区别开
Kastle-Meyer		[医] 卡-麦二氏试验（Kastle-Meyer 血迹反应法是检测血液中的血红素经由氧化还原反应，在数秒内产生颜色反应的测试，可初步筛检检体中是否含有血液）

Notes to the Text

1. The samples in drug analysis are typically pharmaceutical raw materials, finished pharmaceutical products or biological samples like human blood or urine which contain one or more drug substances.

解析：typically pharmaceutical raw materials, finished pharmaceutical products or biological samples… 为平行结构（parallel structure）；which contain one or more drug substances 作为后置定语定语从句修饰名词词组 human blood or urine。

译文：药物分析的样本为药物原材料、成品药物或者生物样本（如含有一种或多种药物成分的人体血液或尿液）。

2. A quantitative analysis, also termed as determination, is intended to measure the exact concentration or the exact amount of the analyte in a given sample.

解析：termed as determination 为动词过去分词短语作定语的用法，相当于 which is termed as；be intended to 意为"打算，意图是"。

译文：量的分析（也被称为定量分析）旨在测定样本中被分析物的精确浓度或精确数量。

3. Paracetamol is the analyte, whereas the rest of tablet, consisting of different pharmaceutical excipients, is the sample matrix.

解析：whereas 连接词，用以比较或对比两个事实，意为"但是，然而，尽管"。whereas 和 while 都可引出表示对比或相反情况的状语从句，两者通常可以换用，但 whereas 语气强并且较书面，语气也较强，通常多位于句中，也可置于句首；while 是普通用语，更为多用。句中 consisting of... 为现在分词做后置定语，相当于定语从句 which consists of 。

译文：对乙酰氨基酚是被分析物，而由不同药用辅料构成的药片其余部分则是样品基质。

4. A flame test, which is an analytic procedure used in chemistry to detect the presence of certain elements, primarily metal ions, based on each element's particular emission spectrum, is also a type of qualitative analysis.

解析：句子的主干为 a flame test is also a type of qualitative analysis；which 引导非限制性定语从句，修饰前面先行词 flame test, used 为过去分词作后置定语，也可看作定语从句 (which is) used... based on each element's particular emission spectrum 为插入语，进行信息的补充和说明，意为"基于每种元素特有的放射光"；based on 表示"基于；以……为基础"。

译文：焰色反应（化学中基于某一成分的发射光谱来检测某种成分是否存在和检测主要金属离子的分析过程）也是一种定性分析。

Post-reading Tasks

I. Answer the following questions according to the text.

1. How does qualitative analysis differ from quantitative analysis?

   _____

2. What is an analyte and what is a sample matrix?

   _____

3. What are typically the samples in drug analysis?

   _____

4. What is the purpose of conducting a flame test?

   _____

II. Complete the following statements with the words or phrases given below. Change the form if necessary.

solution	prior to	distinguish from	numerous	detect
identify	consist of	behavior	amount	transformation

5. He tried to escape_____by disguising himself as an old man.

6. This test_____a number of multiple choice questions.

7. The young lady_____courageously in the face of danger.

8. Any possible_____can only come about through dialogue.

9. His character seems to have undergone a complete_____since his marriage.

10. Although the job takes a significant_____of time, most students agree that the experience is worth it.

11. It is the superior intelligence and the use of language that man other animals.

12. Research suggests that a newly _____gene known as insomniacs (失眠症患者) may play a role in keeping us asleep.

13. They ran into_____difficulties in_____conducting the experiment.

14. All the arrangements should have been completed_____our departure.

III. Read the passage and decide whether the following statements are true (T) or false (F) according to the passage.

The number of abnormal test findings recorded by anti-doping (反兴奋剂) authorities worldwide increased by more than 20% last year, according to a report by the World Anti-Doping Agency.

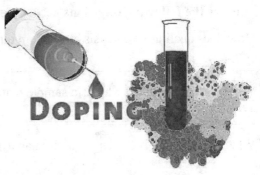

The number of test carried out on the use of doping has increased as compared with last year. There were 5,962 adverse or atypical (非典型的) test results across all sports in 2013, compared with 4,723 in 2012. The number of tests carried out rose by only 0.8% in the same period. In total, 269,878 samples were analyzed across 35 Olympic and 58 non-Olympic sports, compared with 267,645 in 2012.

Among Olympic sports, football, athletics and cycling conducted the most tests, but weightlifting and wrestling had the highest rate of adverse findings. Adverse test results were recorded in sports as diverse as chess, bridge and boccie (地滚球).

Adverse findings are those that detect the presence of a prohibited substance. Atypical findings are those that necessitate further investigation by anti-doping authorities. Atypical findings may correspond to multiple analyses performed on the same athlete.

The increase comes in a year in which sports such as football and tennis stepped up their use of the athlete biological passport programme, which allows authorities to collect and compare biological data and spot discrepancies (差异) over time that suggest possible doping. Other sports, such as cycling, have stiffened the "whereabouts rule" (行踪规则) that requires athletes to provide the authorities with regular information about their location and possible windows for testing.

However, British 800m runner Jenny Meadows says drug-takers in sport are still getting away with it. "People are still taking drugs and always will," she said. The margin of error between coming first and third is so tiny that people will always looks for ways to break that down. "You look at Tyson Gay and Justin Gatlin lining up last week in the 100m (both men have served bans from athletics after failing drugs tests). It makes you feel sick because they are still getting sponsorship and prize money. It's not fair on the rest of us. I do think the sport is being cleaned up and these figures send out a message of 'we'll find you eventually' but unfortunately there are always sophisticated ways to cheat the system."

The report also reveals which national anti-doping authorities test their athletes most frequently. Russia and China lead the way, each testing more than 10,000 samples in 2013. UK Anti-Doping, the body responsible for testing British athletes, analyzed nearly 5,000 samples.

☐ 15. Due to the increase of test on doping, the number of abnormal test findings has decreased as compared with last year.

☐ 16. Only samples for Olympic sports were collected and analyzed this year.

☐ 17. Among Olympic sports, football, athletics and cycling had the highest rate of adverse findings.

☐ 18. No adverse results were found in tests on sports such as chess.

☐ 19. Adverse findings are those in which the presence of a certain banned substance is detected.

☐ 20. More use of athlete biological passport programme in sports like football and tennis has contributed to the increase of abnormal test findings.

☐ 21. Due to stricter ways to detect doping, no drug-taker in sport can get away with it and the system is kept fair to every participant.

☐ 22. Russia and China are the two countries whose anti-doping authorities perform tests on their athletes most frequently worldwide.

药学英语

Practical Writing

Memo

Read and Understand

To: Philip Reater, Laboratory Management
From: Leo Mason, Quality Assurance Internal Auditing
Date: Monday
Subject: Annual audit for laboratory safety

This memo is to advise you that your department has been scheduled for a periodic audit of the laboratory safety systems and procedures.

The timetable for various laboratory audits is as follows:

Laboratory 1: Tuesday and Wednesday

Laboratory 2: Wednesday and Thursday

Laboratory 3: Thursday and Friday

Please make sure that all the laboratory staff are advised and prepared in accordance with standard audit procedure. Our goal is to identify any areas requiring corrective or preventive action. This done to assure compliance with industry standards, especially for safety procedures.

Please confirm receipt of this memo.

L. Mason

Writing Skills

备忘录，也称公务便条，是公司、团体内部各部门之间最普遍的书面交流方式之一。来自英语的 memorandum，实际应用中通常使用其缩写形式 memo，作标题时一定要大写首字母，或者4个字母都大写。

备忘录由名称 (title)，标题区 (heading) 和正文 (body) 三部分组成。其中标题区包括四部分内容：备忘录的撰写人、收件人、发送日期及主题。正文部分不需要加称呼和结束语，直接说明具体内容即可；文字要求明白易懂，不必太正式，也不可过于口语化。

备忘录的基本格式如下（排列格式多为齐头式）：

Memo

To: 写出全名，有时可以加上职位

From: 写出全名，有时可以加上职位

Date: 写出完整日期，月份可以采用缩写

Subject: 主题简短，明确，具体

Body: 直接写出重点，把主要的信息写出来。可以只有一个句子，也可以有好几个段落。

Writing Practice

Write a memo based on the following information.

假设你是销售部经理 John Green，请以 John Green 的名义按以下信息给本公司其他各部门经理写一个内部通知。

主题：讨论 2020 年第一季度药品销售计划

通告时间：2019 年 10 月 20 日

正文内容：本部门已制定 2020 年第一季度的药品销售计划，将于 2019 年 10 月 25 日下午 2:00 在本公司会议室开会讨论这一计划，希望各部门经理前来参会。如不能到会，请提前告知本部门秘书。

Memo

To: _____

From: _____

Date: _____

Subject: _____

_____

_____

_____

_____

_____

_____

Grammar

Past Participle Used as Attribute
过去分词作定语

1. 过去分词短语作后置定语

过去分词短语作后置定语，具有被动和完成意义。在语态上，表被动；在时间上，表示动作已经发生或完成，与它所修饰的名词有逻辑（意义）上的动宾关系。

The books, written by Mo Yan, are very popular with Chinese readers.

莫言写的书很受中国读者的欢迎。

French is one of the major languages used at international meetings.

法语是国际会议上（被）使用的主要语言之一。

名词 book 与动词 write 之间、名词 languages 和动词 use 之间的关系为被动关系，所以分别需要过去分词 written、used 来做后置定语进行修饰，表示逻辑上的被动关系。

2. 过去分词作后置定语及前置定语

过去分词既可以作后置定语，也可以前置。过去分词短语作定语通常后置，单个的过去分词作定语通常作前置定语。

（1）过去分词短语作定语时，通常放在被修饰的名词之后，它的作用相当于一个定语从句。

This will be the best novel of its kind ever written (=that has ever been written).

这将是这类小说中写得最好的。

Who were the so-called guests invited (=who had been invited) to your party last night?

昨晚被邀请参加你的晚会的那些客人是谁呀？

The techniques of this science are used to identify the substances which may be present in a material and to determine the exact amounts of the identified substance.

这门科学技术被用来确定物体中可能存在的物质并测定已确定物质的精确含量。

Analytical chemistry is a scientific discipline used to study the chemical composition, structure and behavior of matter.

分析化学是一门研究物质化学成分、结构和行为的学科。

（2）单个的过去分词作定语，通常放在被修饰的名词之前，表示被动和完成意义，相当于一个形容词。

A 类：被动意义

an honored guest 一位受尊敬的客人

The injured workers are now being taken good care of in the hospital.

受伤的工人现正在医院受到良好的照料。

B 类：完成意义

a retired teacher 一位退休的教师

They are cleaning the fallen leaves in the yard.

他们正在打扫院子里的落叶。

Exercises

I. Rewrite the following sentences using past participle phrases.

1. Is this the book that is recommended by your teacher?
   _____

2. Hangzhou, which is known to the world for its West Lake, is one of the most beautiful cities in China.
   _____

3. All the windows that were broken yesterday have been repaired.
   _____

4. The guns that had been stolen from the police station were found in the forest.
   _____

II. Complete the following sentences by using past participle as attributive.

5. Many people believe the English_____（在电视和收音机上说的）is standard English.

6. The problem _____（在昨天会议上讨论的）was

very difficult to solve.

7. The students _____ (受到老师鼓舞的) worked harder than ever before.

8. Mary is a new nurse and her job is to take care of the _____ (受伤的) soldiers.

9. Five people won the award, a title _____ (授予普通人的) for their contributions to environmental protections.

III. **Translate a passage from Chinese into English and try to use at least one past participle phrase as attributive in your translation.**

华佗（约公元145～208)是中国古代一位著名的医生，生活在汉代和三国时期。华佗是中国历史上进行麻醉手术的第一人。他因手术和麻醉的知识被世人尊重，也因针灸、中草药和医疗实践方面的能力为人熟知。此外，基于对五种动物，即虎、鹿、熊、猿、鸟的研究，华佗创编了被称为"五禽戏"的疗法和健身方法，成为中国民间最受欢迎的健身方法之一。

参考词汇：

三国时期 the Three Kingdoms Period；麻醉手术 anaesthesia operation；针灸 acupuncture；五禽戏 "Wuqinxi" or "Exercise of the Five Animals"

_____

_____

_____

_____

_____

Have Some Fun

Bianque was a famous physician in ancient China. One day the King of Wei asked him, "You and your two brothers are all skilled in medicine, which of you is the best?"

Bianque answered, "My eldest brother is the best, the next is my second brother, and the last is me." The King asked again, "Then how is it that you are the most famous?" Bianque replied, "My eldest brother treats a disease when it is just beginning to show symptoms (症状). What he does is to remove the pathogen (病原，病原体) —members of my family can all see that but other people cannot. That's why he doesn't enjoy wide recognition. My second brother cures a disease in its early stages. People thus mistake him as only capable of treating minor illnesses. So he is merely known within this locality and its neighborhood. As for me, I treat a disease when it is already well developed and very serious. People observe me perform bloodletting by injecting tubes into vessels or applying medical ointment (药膏) on the skin, and thus look upon me as well-versed (通晓的，精通的) in medicine. So I have become well-known all over the country."

The King was quite satisfied and said, "You've given an excellent explanation."

What we can learn from the story is this: Prevention is better than control, which in turn is better than remedy after the event.

Unit 4 Herbal Medicine

Lead-in

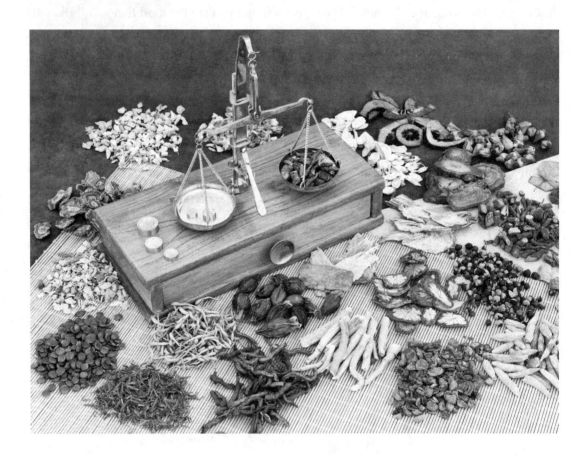

Herbal medicine has been used for a long time to treat a variety of diseases from simple cold, headache, and stomachache to serious diseases such as pneumonia, hemorrhage, food poison and tuberculosis. Do you know anything more about herbal medicine? Read texts in this unit carefully and find out the answer to the question.

Unit 4 Herbal Medicine

Speaking and Listening

Dialogue

Good Medicine Tastes Bitter

Susan: Morning, Hong! What are you drinking? Smells bitter!

Li Hong: Morning, Susan. This is traditional Chinese herbal medicine. My throat hurts for a week. I hope this herbal medicine will work.

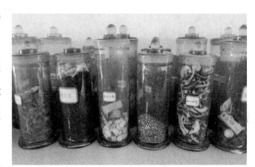

Susan: Oh, I'm sorry to hear that. Don't worry. Your throat will surely heal (痊愈). By the way, are all Chinese medicines so bitter?

Li Hong: Good medicine for health tastes bitter to the mouth. (良药苦口利于病。) Generally speaking, they are. However, the degree of bitterness is different. Some are even a little sweet.

Susan: That's good! Oh, my grandma always has a backache. I really want to bring some traditional Chinese medicine for her to try. Is that possible?

Li Hong: Well, The herbal medicine is usually taken in the form of a "recipe" called a prescription. The TCM practitioner (医师) has to diagnose the patient to make up a prescription.

Susan: I get it. My grandma must see a TCM practitioner in person. Thank you!

Start New Dialogue

★ Discuss and role-play a conversation with your partner based on the given information.

   As a TCM practitioner, you are invited to give a presentation entitled Traditional Chinese Medicine in an International Conference on Pharmaceutical Sciences.

Stick Up Your Ears

★ Listen to the recording and fill in the blanks according to what you hear.

   Headaches can (1)_____ in a variety of disease patterns in traditional Chinese medicine. Some headaches are (2)_____ with external pernicious (有害的) influences, such as wind cold, wind heat, or wind damp. Others occur as a symptom of internal (3)_____, such as liver fire, blood stagnation, *qi* deficiency (气虚), or blood deficiency (血亏). It is especially important to have an (4)_____ diagnosis when treating a headache, since the wrong treatment can actually make the condition (5)_____.

When a headache is caused by an external pernicious influence, it can occur suddenly, often along with other symptoms of wind. When it is due to wind cold, the pain is (6)_____ in the back or the top of the head. Other symptoms could be an aversion to cold (畏寒), tight and sore shoulders and neck, and nasal congestion (鼻塞). The classic formula for this pattern is Chuanxiong Chatiao Wan (川芎茶调丸) taken with warm water. When it is due to wind heat, the headache can be quite (7)_____. Other symptoms may be fever, sore throat, thirst, and a floating, rapid pulse. In this case, the appropriate formula is Yinqiao Jiedu Pian or Ganmaoling Granules.

A (8)_____ internal cause of headache is liver *yang* rising up to the head, which may occur when a person (9) _____ anger or frustration, or it can be a result of long-term deficiency of liver *yin*. Symptoms are dizziness, irritability (易怒), and nausea; the headache is a throbbing pain on the sides of the head or behind the eyes. The classic formula for this condition is Tianma Gouteng Yin, which is also quite (10)_____ in relieving tight neck and shoulders that can accompany the headache.

Reading and Writing

In-depth Reading

Herbal Medicine

Do you know that about 25 percent of the drugs prescribed worldwide are derived from plants? Of the 252 drugs in the World Health Organization's essential medicine list, 11 percent are exclusively of plant origin. In fact, about 200 years ago the first pharmacological

Unit 4 Herbal Medicine

compound, morphine, was produced from opium extracted from the seed pods of the poppy flower.

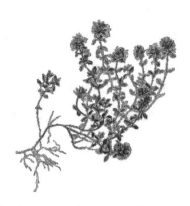

Since then, scientists have been studying plants to create the pharmaceutical products we know today. But after years of overmedicating, facing resistant bacteria in the microbiome and treating the illness rather than the root of the problem, people are beginning to pay more attention to natural, herbal medicine.

Herbal medicines are naturally occurring, plant-derived substances that are used to treat illnesses within local or regional healing practices. These products are complex mixtures of organic chemicals that may come from any raw or processed part of a plant.

Herbal medicine has its roots in every culture around the world. There are many different systems of traditional medicine, and the philosophy and practices of each are influenced by social conditions, environment and geographic location, but these systems all agree on a holistic approach to life. Well-known systems of herbal medicine like Traditional Chinese Medicine and Ayurvedic Medicine believe in the central idea that there should be an emphasis on health rather than on disease. By using healing herbs, people can thrive and focus on their overall conditions, rather than on a particular ailment that typically arises from a lack of equilibrium of the mind, body and environment.

Although botanical medicine has been practiced for thousands of years, it continues to be of use in the modern, Western world. The World Health Organization recently estimated that 80 percent of people worldwide rely on herbal medicines for some part of their primary health care, and the worldwide annual market for these products is approaching $60 billion. People in the United States have become more interested in herbal medicine because of the rising cost of prescription medication and the returning interest in natural or organic remedies.

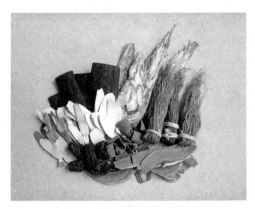

Whole herbs contain many ingredients that are used to treat diseases and relieve symptoms. Herbal medicine, also called botanical medicine, uses the plant's seeds, berries, roots, leaves, bark or flowers for medicinal purposes. The biological properties of these plants have beneficial effects.

Other factors are responsible for their benefits as well, such as the type of environment in which the plant grew, the way in which it was harvested and how it was processed. The plant is either sold raw or as extracts, where it's macerated with water, alcohol or other solvents to extract some of the chemicals. The resulting products contain dozens of chemicals, including fatty acids, sterols, alkaloids, flavonoids, glycosides, saponins and others.

(461 words)

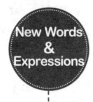

herbal /ˈhɜːbl/	adj.	草药的；草本的
	n.	植物志；草本书
morphine /ˈmɔːfiːn/	n.	[药] 吗啡
opium /ˈəʊpɪəm/	n.	鸦片；麻醉剂
	adj.	鸦片的
poppy /ˈpɒpɪ/	n.	罂粟花，罂粟属植物；深红色
	adj.	罂粟科的
holistic /həˈlɪstɪk/	adj.	整体的；全盘的
ailment /ˈeɪlmənt/	n.	小病；不安
equilibrium /ˌiːkwɪˈlɪbrɪəm/	n.	均衡；平静；保持平衡的能力
botanical /bəˈtænɪkl/	adj.	植物学的
	n.	植物性药材
sterol /ˈstɪərɒl/	n.	[有化] 甾醇；固醇
flavonoid /ˈfleɪvənɔɪd/	n.	黄酮类；[有化] 类黄酮
glycoside /ˈglaɪkəˌsaɪd/	n.	配糖体；配糖类
saponin /ˈsæpənɪn/	n.	肥皂精；[生化] 皂素
since then		从那时起
rather than		而不是；宁可……也不愿
has its roots in		根源于
agree on		与……达成一致
be responsible for		对……负责任
dozens of		几十；许多
Ayurvedic Medicine		印度式草药疗法（世界上最古老的医疗系统之一）

Notes to the Text

1. In fact, about 200 years ago the first pharmacological compound, morphine, was produced from opium extracted from the seed pods of the poppy flower.

解析：was produced from 被动语态，意为"由……制成"；extracted from 动词过去分词短语作定语，可译为"从……中提取"。

译文：事实上，大约200年前，第一种药用化合物吗啡就是从罂粟花的种子荚中提取出来的。

2. But after years of overmedicating, facing resistant bacteria in the microbiome and treating the illness rather than the root of the problem, people are beginning to pay more attention to natural, herbal medicine.

解析：facing... and treating... 非谓语动词现在分词短语作原因状语；pay more attention to 为动词短语，意指"更多地关注……"。

译文：然而多年过度用药后，面对微生物群中耐药细菌的出现，疾病也只是治疗而不是从病源上解决问题，人们开始将更多的注意力转向天然草药。

3. There are many different systems of traditional medicine, and the philosophy and practices of each are influenced by social conditions, environment and geographic location, but these systems all agree on a holistic approach to life.

解析：are influenced by 动词短语，意为"受到……的影响"；agree on 意为"在……方面达成一致意见或达成共识"。

译文：传统医学有许多不同的体系，每种体系的理论和实践都受到社会条件、环境和地理位置的影响，但这些体系都认同将生命视作一个整体。

4. Well-known systems of herbal medicine like Traditional Chinese Medicine and Ayurvedic Medicine believe in the central idea that there should be an emphasis on health rather than on disease.

解析：...idea that... 为同位语从句，that 引导的名词性从句是 idea 的同位语。

译文：世界闻名的中草药体系，如传统中医和印度中医，都认同这样一个中心思想：医学应当重在关注健康、预防疾病，而不是一味地治疗疾病。

5. Other factors are responsible for their benefits as well, such as the type of environment in which the plant grew, the way in which it was harvested and how it was processed.

解析：are responsible for 意为"对……负责"或"是……的原因"；as well 为副词短语，表示"也，同样地"。

译文：这些植物生物特性的益处也与其他因素有关，如植物生长的环境、收获的方式以及加工的方式。

Post-reading Tasks

I. Answer the following questions according to the text.

1. Why do people begin to pay more attention to herbal medicine?
   _____

2. What is the central idea believed by Traditional Chinese Medicine and Ayurvedic Medicine?
   _____

3. Why do people in the United States become more interested in herbal medicine?
   _____

4. What are the factors responsible for the benefits of plants?
   _____

II. Complete the following statements with the words given below. Change the form if necessary.

| holistic | herbal | equilibrium | botanical | ailment |
| benefit | responsible | root | agree | extract |

5. A doctor should be _____ for the lives of the patients.

6. _____ Medicine, which includes Oriental Medicine is based upon evaluation of and treatment of these four components.

7. The two countries have not reached _____ on the issues discussed.

8. Every mammal on this planet instinctively develops a natural _____ with the surrounding environment.

9. He was examined again and then prescribed a different _____ medicine.

10. In India, mathematics has its_____ in Vedic literature which is nearly 4,000 years old.

11. The most effective new _____ are extracts from cola nut and marine algae.

12. I don't have even the slightest _____.

13. They have invested in _____ of internet firms around the globe.

14. This substance is _____ from seaweed.

III. Read the passage with ten blanks. You are required to select one word for each blank from a list of choices given in a word bank following the passage. You may not use the words in the blank more than once.

A few months ago, I was down with a terrible cold which ended in a persistent bad cough. No matter how many different (15)____ I tried, I still couldn't get rid of the cough Not only did it (16)____ my teaching but also my life as a whole Then one day after class, a student came up to me and (17)____ traditional Chinese medicine. From her description, Chinese medicine sounded as if it had magic power that worked wonders. I was (18)____ because I knew so little about it and have never tried it before. Eventually, my cough got so much (19)____ that I couldn't sleep at night, so I decided to give it a try. The Chinese doctor took my pulse and asked to see my tongue, both of which were new (20)____ to me because they are both non-existent in Western medicine. Then the doctor gave me a scraping (刮) treatment known as "Gua Sha". I was a little (21)____ at first because he used a smooth edged tool to scrape the skin on my neck and shoulders A few minutes later, the (22)____ strokes started to produce a relieving effect and my body and mind began to (23)____ deeper into relaxation. I didn't feel any improvement in my condition in the first couple of days, but after a few more regular visits to the doctor, my cough started to (24)_____. Then within a matter of weeks, it was completely gone!

(A) deepen (B) experiences (C) hesitant (D) inconvenience (E) lessen
(F) licenses (G) pressured (H) recommended (I) remedies (J) scared
(K) sensitive (L) sink (M) temporary (N) tremble (O) worse

Practical Writing

Bar Chart

Read and Understand

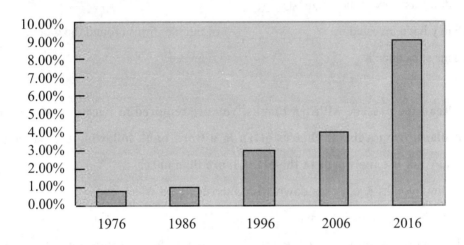

In recent years China has experienced a dramatic increase in the divorce rate. According to the chart, during the last decade, the divorce rate in big cities has increased as much as it had in the previous thirty years.

The upward trend in divorce seems to be a mirror of some important changes in Chinese society. First, legal changes have simplified divorce procedures, and removed barriers to divorce. More and more people, both young and old, are now benefiting from, even taking advantage of the new law which for the first time in history allows a couple to get divorced merely for love's sake.

Second, there has been a significant change in social attitude towards the divorced persons. The act of divorce is no longer considered a social stigma (耻辱). Finally, the change in personal economic activities may also facilitate (助长) divorce. The unprecedented (前所未有的) social mobility in the last 10 years both within the country and across the land has placed severe strains on married couples, not only in terms of geographic separation, but also psychological change.

Whatever changes leading to the rise in divorce rates, the fact and the statistics alone reflect the change in people's traditional view of marriage and family life.

Useful Information

A bar chart is a graphic representation of project activities, shown in a time-scaled bar line. There are many disadvantages of bar charts, such as simplicity, duration of each activity, intelligibility. Basically, with a bar chart, you need to describe the bars and their values. When describing a bar chart you first have to decide in what order to describe the bars, highest value to lowest value or lowest value to highest value. It may be a mixture of this. If there are very many bars, you can sometimes group together 2 or 3 bars which have similar or the same values. If there are very many and you can't group them, then just describe the ones that are the most significant.

Some useful expressions:

The bar chart illustrates that... 该柱状图展示了……

The graph provides some interesting data regarding...
该图为我们提供了有关……的有趣数据。

As is shown/demonstrated/exhibited in the diagram/graph/chart/table...
如图所示……

As can be seen from the chart, great changes have taken place in...
从图中可以看出，……发生了巨大变化。

Over the period from... to... the... remained level.
在……至……期间，……基本不变。

Writing Practice

Write an essay titled "Traditional Chinese Medicine (TCM) Exports" based on the following chart.

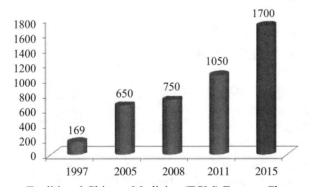

Traditional Chinese Medicine (TCM) Exports Chart

You should start your essay with a brief description of the picture and then express your views on Traditional Chinese medicine (TCM).

_____
_____
_____
_____
_____

Grammar

Passive Voice
被动语态

英语有两种语态：主动语态和被动语态。主动语态表示句子的主语是谓语动词的执行者；被动语态表示主语是谓语动作的承受者。

1. 构成

（1）助动词 be + 过去分词。

（2）情态动词 + be + 过去分词。

2. 主动语态与被动语态之间的转换

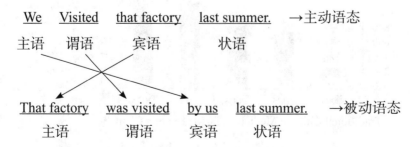

3. 被动语态的时态变化

	Be	Past Participle	Tense
The butter	is	kept here.	Present simple
The window	was	broken.	Past simple
The work	will be	done soon.	Future simple
The bridge	is being	repaired.	Present continuous
The cheese	was being	eaten by mice.	Past continuous
Our work	has been	finished.	Present perfect
The car	hadn't been	used much.	Past perfect
The house	will have been	built by then.	Future perfect

4. 被动语态的使用情境

(1) 施动者未知或不重要。

Our car was stolen last night.

昨晚，我们的车被偷了。

(2) 施动者众所周知。

Cameron was sacked last week.

卡梅伦上周被解雇了。

(3) 用于描述客观事实。

The lasagna is baked in an oven for 35 minutes at 250 degrees Celsius.

千层面在250℃的烤箱里烤35分钟。

(4) 用于新闻报道或给出指令。

Five people were arrested at a nightclub last night.

昨晚有五人在一家夜总会被捕。

Exercises

I. Rewrite the following sentences using passive voice.

1. All the students who are applying for the government loan must observe this rule.

2. The sad story needn't have caused him so much distress.

3. People would never forget the accident.

4. People are building a new bridge now.

II. Read the following statements carefully, and tick the passive voices.

☐ 5. The people present at the meeting were annoyed with the tedious speech.

☐ 6. The people who wanted to attend the meeting were surprised by the announcement of the adjournment without day.

☐ 7. The houses were beautifully decorated.

☐ 8. The houses were decorated and rented to those who were badly in need of shelters.

☐ 9. The book is not illustrated.

☐ 10. The book was illustrated by a famous artist.

☐ 11. I'm interested in my own hobbies, such as collecting stamps, raising birds and fishing.

☐ 12. I was interested by what you showed me.

☐ 13. I shall be much obliged to you for an early reply.

☐ 14. The house will get white-washed next week.

III. Translate a passage from Chinese into English and try to use the passive voice if possible.

针灸是中医学的重要组成部分。按照中医的经络理论，针灸疗法主要是通过疏通经络、调和气血，来达到阴阳平衡，使肝脏趋于调和之目的。其特点是内病外治。主要疗法是用针刺入病人身体的特定穴位，或用艾火的温热刺激烧灼病人穴位，以达到刺激经络、治疗病痛的目的。针灸以其独特的优势，流传至今并享誉海外，与中餐、功夫、中药一起被誉为中国的"新四大国粹"。

参考词汇：

针灸 acupuncture； 经络 meridian； 穴位 acupuncture point； 国粹 the quintessence of Chinese culture

_____

_____

_____

_____

_____

Have Some Fun

Sun Simiao (581 ~ 682), born in Huayuan Tongchuang city, Shaanxi Province today, was a medical expert of China in Tang Dynasty. His book, *Qianjin Yaofang* (*Essential Formulas Worth a Thousand Ducats*), listed more than 8,000 recipes of medicines, which was used for medicinal purposes, and applied to food therapy and health maintenance as well. This book is honored as the earliest clinical medical encyclopedia in China, which earned him the title as Yaowang (China's King of Medicine) for his significant contributions to Chinese medicine. His masterpiece work, *Da Yi Jing Cheng* (*On the Absolute Sincerity of Great Physicians*), which is also known as "the Chinese Hippocratic Oath", came straight to the point that a doctor should have both consummate medical skills and high-spirited medical ethics. He was the founder of Chinese medical ethics thoughts.

Unit 5 Drug Label

Lead-in

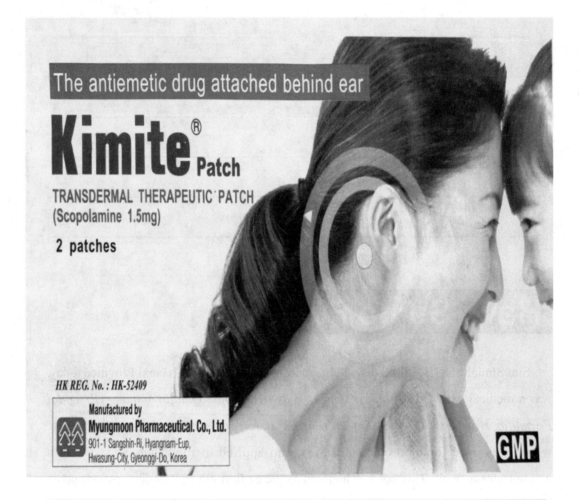

> Although medicines can make you feel better and help you get well, it's important to know that ALL medicines, both prescription and over-the-counter, have risks as well as benefits. It's a must to have a careful look at the drug label before you use any medicine.

Speaking and Listening

Dialogue

At the Pharmacy (1)

Patient: Excuse me, is it the Pharmacy?

Pharmacist: Yes, madam. What can I do for you?

Patient: I have a terrible cold. Apart from that, I have a headache. Can you suggest something I can take to relieve the pain?

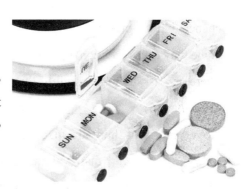

Pharmacist: Don't you have a prescription?

Patient: No, I haven't gone to see a doctor.

Pharmacist: Are you allergic to any type of medication?

Patient: I don't know exactly. I think that I can take most drugs.

Pharmacist: (picks up a small box) I recommend this brand for quick relief.

Patient: Will this really help?

Pharmacist: According to the label, yes.

Patient: How do I take it?

Pharmacist: Please take 2 tablets each time, 3 times a day after meals.

Patient: Are there any side effects?

Pharmacist: It will make you feel sleepy, so don't drive a car after taking it.

Patient: Thank you for reminding me.

Pharmacist: You're welcome. I hope you will recover soon.

Start New Dialogue

★ Discuss and role-play a conversation with your partner based on the given information.

You are a pharmacist at a pharmacy. A foreign patient comes to buy some medicines. You will give some recommendations and talk to the foreign patient on the usage of the medicines.

Stick Up Your Ears

★ Listen to the recording and fill in the blanks according to what you hear.

There are several (1)_____ of risks from medicine use: the possibility of a (2)_____ interaction between the medicine and a food, beverage, dietary supplement (including vitamins and herbals), or another medicine. (Combinations of any of these products could (3)_____ the chance that there may be interactions.); the chance that the medicine may not work as (4)_____. the possibility that the medicine may cause additional problems. For example, every time you (5)_____ a car, there are risks—the possibility that unwanted or unexpected things could happen. You could have an (6)_____, causing costly damage to your car, or injury to yourself or a loved one. But there are also benefits to riding in a car: you can travel farther and (7)_____ than walking, bring home more groceries from the store, and travel in cold or wet weather in greater comfort. To obtain the (8)_____ of riding in a car, you think through the risks. You consider the condition of your car and the road, (9)_____, before deciding to make that trip to the store. The same is true before using any medicine. Every choice to (10)_____ involves thinking through the helpful effects as well as the possible unwanted effects.

Reading and Writing

In-depth Reading

Always Read the Label

In the United States, each OTC (over-the-counter medicine) has a Drug Facts label. The Drug Facts label is there to help you choose the right OTC medicine and use it safely. All medicines, even OTC medicines, can cause side effects (unwanted or unexpected effects). But if the directions on the label are followed, the chance of side effects can be lowered.

Reading the product label is the most important part of taking care of yourself or your

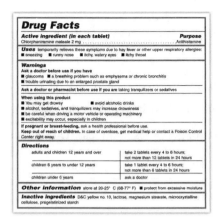

family when using OTC medicines (available without a prescription). The OTC medicine label has always contained important usage and safety information for consumers, but now that information will be more consistent and even easier to read and to understand.

The U.S. Food and Drug Administration has issued a regulation to make sure the labels on all OTC medicines (from a tube of fluoride toothpaste to a bottle of cough syrup) have information listed in the same order; are arranged in a simpler eye-catching, consistent style; and may contain words easier to understand.

Below is an example of what the new OTC medicine label looks like.

The **Active ingredients/Purpose** section tells you the part of the medicine that makes it work (active ingredient), what it does (purpose), and how much of each active ingredient is in each unit (such as pill, capsule, or teaspoon). Choose a medicine that treats only the problem(s) you want to treat. Extra medicine won't help, and could cause harmful or unwanted side effects.

The **Uses** section tells you the problems the medicine will treat. The problem(s) you want to treat should match at least one of the Uses.

The **Warnings** section tells you:

• when to talk to a doctor first;

• how the medicine might make a person feel;

• when the medicine shouldn't be used;

• things that shouldn't be done while using the medicine;

• when to stop using the medicine;

• to check with a doctor before using medicine if the person is pregnant or breastfeeding;

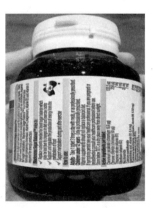

• to keep medicines away from children.

The **Directions** section tells you how to use the medicine safely:

• how much to use;

• how to use it;

• how often to use it (how many times per day, how many hours apart);

• how long it can be used.

The **Other information** section tells you how to keep the medicine when it isn't being used.

The **Inactive ingredients** section tells you the parts of the medicine that aren't the active ingredient(s). These parts are added to the active ingredient(s) to help shape the form, to flavor or color the medicine, or to help the medicine last longer (preservatives). Check this section to see if there is anything that might cause an allergic reaction.

(468 words)

New Words & Expressions

label /ˈleɪbl/	n.	标签；标记；商标
prescription /prɪˈskrɪpʃn/	n.	[医] 药方，处方；处方药
contain /kənˈteɪn/	vt.	包含；容纳；含有，包括
usage /ˈjuːsɪdʒ/	n.	用途
consistent /kənˈsɪstənt/	adj.	一致的；连续的；不矛盾的
administration /ədˌmɪnɪˈstreɪʃn/	n.	管理；实行；(政府) 行政机关
regulation /ˌregjuˈleɪʃn/	n.	规则；法规，规章；管制
fluoride /ˈflɔːraɪd/	n.	[化] 氟化物
toothpaste /ˈtuːθpeɪst/	n.	牙膏
syrup /ˈsɪrəp/	n.	糖浆，糖汁；糖浆类药品
list /lɪst/	vt.	列出，列入；把……编列成表；记入名单内
ingredient /ɪnˈɡriːdiənt/	n.	(混合物的) 组成部分；(烹调的) 原料；（构成）要素，因素
pill /pɪl/	n.	药丸；弹丸
capsule /ˈkæpsjuːl/	n.	胶囊
teaspoon /ˈtiːspuːn/	n.	茶匙；一茶匙的量
treat /triːt/	v.	对待；治疗；处理；款待
match /mætʃ/	vt.	相配；适应；使较量；使等同于
pregnant /ˈpreɡnənt/	adj.	怀孕的；充溢着……
breastfeed /ˈbrestfiːd/	v.	用母乳喂养，哺乳
inactive /ɪnˈæktɪv/	adj.	不活动的，不活跃的

flavor /ˈfleɪvə/	vt.	给……调味；给……增添风趣
last /lɑːst/	vi.	持续
preservative /prɪˈzɜːvətɪv/	n.	防腐剂；防护剂
allergic /əˈlɜːdʒɪk/	adj.	过敏的；过敏症的
drug facts		药品说明
side effects		副作用；不良作用
active ingredient		有效成分，活性成分

Notes to the Text

1. But if the directions on the label are followed, the chance of side effects can be lowered.

解析：此句的主句和从句都用的被动语态；follow one's advice/direction/order… 为固定搭配。

译文：按照标签上的说明去做，引起副作用的概率就会降低。

2. The U.S. Food and Drug Administration has issued a regulation to make sure the labels on all OTC medicines (from a tube of fluoride toothpaste to a bottle of cough syrup) have information listed in the same order; are arranged in a simpler eye-catching, consistent style; and may contain words easier to understand.

解析：to make sure…to understand 是动词不定式短语作目的状语，其中含有一个带三个并列谓语的宾语从句：have, are arranged, and may contain；listed in the same order 是 information 的宾语补足语；easier to understand 为 words 的后置定语。

译文：美国食品药品监督管理局规定：所有非处方药上的标签（从含氟牙膏到瓶装止咳糖浆）必须做到信息要以同样的顺序列出，要以更简单、醒目、一致的风格排列并使用简洁易懂的文字。

3. The problem(s) you want to treat should match at least one of the Uses.

解析：you want to treat 是 problem 的后置定语，起限定修饰作用。

译文：你要治疗的病症应该至少符合药品说明标签上"适应证"的一种。

4. These parts are added to the active ingredient(s) to help shape the form, to flavor or color the medicine, or to help the medicine last longer (preservatives).

解析：flavor 和 color 均为及物动词；to help…, to flavor or color…, or to help… 为平行结构（parallel structure）。

译文：在有效成分中加入这些非活性成分是为了帮助药品成形、调味或上色，或使药品保存更久。

Post-reading Tasks

I. Answer the following questions according to the text.

1. What can drug facts labels do for customers?
   _____

2. What does the Active ingredients/Purpose section tell the users?
   _____

3. What requirements must drug labels meet, according to the regulation issued by FDA?
   _____

4. Why do we need to check the Inactive ingredient section?
   _____

II. Complete the following statements with the words or phrases given below. Change the form if necessary.

| side effects | in the same order | last | prescription | issue |
| allergic reaction | eye-catching | match | consistent | flavor |

5. The government_____a statement to prevent the rumor from spreading.

6. The child is allergic to animal hair, for he has_____ every time he contacts dogs or cats.

7. The beef smells strongly_____ with pepper.

8. We'd better consult a doctor before using a drug, because even OTC medicines have _____.

Unit 5 Drug Label

9. Do put the books_____ as before after you read them.

10. While making a post, you should think to make it_____ first.

11. How many hours will the meeting _____?

12. After the doctor wrote the _____ for me, he told me how to use the medicines in detail.

13. What you say now is not _____ with what you said last week.

14. I think her hair style _____ her face very well.

III. Read the following passage carefully and choose the best answer.

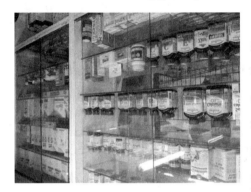

American medicine cabinets contain a growing choice of nonprescription, over-the-counter (OTC) medicines to treat an expanding range of ailments. OTC medicines often do more than relieve aches, pains and itches. Some can prevent diseases like tooth decay, cure diseases like athlete's foot and, with a doctor's guidance, help manage recurring conditions like virus infection, migraine (偏头痛) and minor pain in arthritis. The U.S. Food and Drug Administration (FDA) determines whether medicines are prescription or nonprescription. The term prescription (Rx) refers to medicines that are safe and effective when used under a doctor's care. Nonprescription or OTC drugs are medicines FDA decides are safe and effective for use without a doctor's prescription. FDA also has the authority to decide when a prescription drug is safe enough to be sold directly to consumers over the counter. This regulatory process allowing Americans to take a more active role in their health care is known as Rx-to-OTC switch. As a result of this process, more than 700 products sold over the counter today use ingredients or dosage strengths available only by prescription 30 years ago. Increased access to OTC medicines is especially important for the maturing population. Two out of three older Americans rate their health as excellent to good, but four out of five report at least one chronic condition. Fact is, today's OTC medicines offer greater opportunity to treat more of the aches and illnesses most likely to appear in our later years. As we live longer, work longer, and take a more active role in our own health care, the need grows to become better informed about <u>self-care</u>. The best way to become better informed—for young and old alike—is to read and understand the information on OTC labels. Next to the medicine itself, label comprehension is the most important part of self-care with OTC medicines. With new opportunities in self-medication come new responsibilities and an increased need for knowledge.

15. The underlined word "self-care" in the article means _____.

    A. patients take care of themselves

    B. patients care about their illnesses

    C. patients buy and use medicines to treat their illnesses without going to see a doctor

    D. patients use medicines prescribed by their doctor by themselves

16. According to the article, which statement is right?

    A. There are more and more OTC medicines today than before.

    B. There are more than 700 OTC medicines on American medicine cabinets.

    C. Doctors can decide which is a prescription or nonprescription drug.

    D. Prescriptions drugs can't be switch to nonprescription drugs.

17. Increased access to OTC medicines is especially important for the_____.

    A. grown-up people

    B. older people

    C. people in good health

    D. older people with chronic illnesses

18. The author of the article intends mainly to tell us that_____.

    A. the differences between prescription drugs and OTC drugs

    B. OTC drugs can treat more and more ailments

    C. self-care improve people's active role in their life

    D. with increased access to OTC drugs, it's the most important to read and understand the information on OTC labels

Practical Writing

A Prescription

Read and Understand

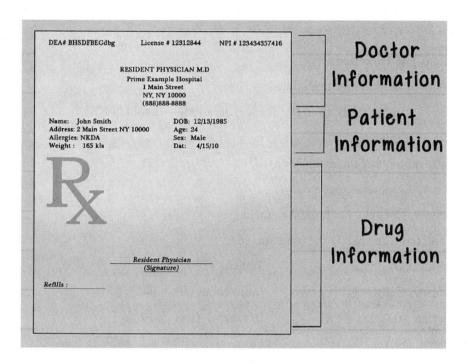

Useful Information

A prescription is an instruction from a prescriber to a dispenser. There is no global standard for prescriptions and every country has its own regulations. Generally speaking, there are basic information, inscription, dispensing directions and patient use directions in a prescription, which should include:

1. Basic Information

* Name, address of prescriber
* Name, address, age of patient
* Date of the prescription
* Signature or initials of prescriber

2. Inscription

* Drug name — can be generic or trade name

* Drug strength — especially if the drug comes in more than one strength

* Drug formulation

3. Dispensing Directions

* Dosage form (bottle size, ointment tube size, or number of tablets or capsules)

* Total amount to be given at the pharmacy and number of refills (preceded by "dispense" "disp" or " # ")

4. Patient Use Directions

* Amount of drug to take each time

* When to take the medication (frequency, duration) — avoid "PRN"

* Route of administration

* How to administer the medication

* When to discontinue use

* Diagnosis (optional but helpful to include)

Common terms to specify the route include:

By mouth (PO) 口服	Topical (TP) 外用
Intramuscular (IM) 肌肉注射	Intravenous (IV) 静脉注射
Intradermal (ID) 皮内注射	Intranasal (IN) 鼻内给药
Sublingual (SL) 舌下给药	Per rectum (PR) 直肠给药

Common expressions to indicate the frequency include:

Twice a day (BID) 一日 2 次	Three times a day (TID) 一日 3 次
Four times a day (QID) 一日 4 次	Every bedtime (QHS) 睡前

Every four hours (Q4H) 每隔 4 个小时

Every four to six hours (Q4-6H) 每隔 4~6 小时

Every week (QWK) 每周

In two of three divided doses 分为 2 或 3 次

A few common examples for special instructions include:

Take with food	饭后服用
Avoid alcohol	避免饮酒
Keep refrigerated	冷藏
Do not freeze	不可冷冻
For external use only	仅限外用
Shake before instillation	注入前摇一摇

Unit 5 Drug Label

Writing Practice

Write a prescription based on the following information.

Lynn J. Orange, 70 years old. Moderate congestive cardiac failure. For several years on digoxin 0.25mg 1 tablet daily. She phones to ask for a repeat prescription. As you have not seen her for some time you ask her to call. During the visit she complains of slight nausea and loss of appetite. No vomiting or diarrhoea. You suspect side effects of digoxin, and call her cardiologist. As she has an appointment with him next week, and he is very busy, he advises you to halve the dose until then.

Prescription:

Robert, Morgan MD
123 Fifth Street
Los Angeles, CA90002

Tel: 112-2235   Fax: 112-2235

Name: Lynn J. Orange   Age:_____

Address: 303 First Street, Los Angeles, CA90035   Date:_____

Rx

Refills: _____

Signature of Prescriber:_____

Grammar

Interrogative + Infinitive
"疑问词 + 不定式"的用法

"疑问词 + 不定式"的用法可以看作名词性从句的简化形式，因其短小精悍、言简意赅而得到广泛应用。

1. 作宾语

(1) 当主句谓语动词是 know, learn, remember, forget, tell, teach, decide, wonder 等，且主句主语与从句主语一致时，宾语从句可简化为"疑问词 + 不定式"结构，或后带双宾语。

She has forgotten how she can open the window. → She has forgotten how to open the window.

她忘记了怎么开窗户。

Could you tell me how I can get to the station? → Could you tell me how to get to the station?

你能告诉我怎么去车站吗？

(2) 也可以在某些介词后作宾语。

They discussed the question of where they would build up the factory. → They discussed the question of where to build up the factory.

他们讨论了在何处建工厂的问题。

I haven't decided on which shirt I will choose, the yellow or the white. → I haven't decided on which shirt to choose, the yellow or the white.

我还没决定选哪件衬衫，黄色的还是白色的。

2. 作主语

What we will do next is still unknown. → What to do next is still unknown.

下一步做什么还不知道。

It doesn't matter now whether we will stay or leave. → It doesn't matter now whether to stay or to leave.

我们是去是留现在无关紧要。

3. 作表语

The problem is where we can get the fund we need. → The problem is where to get the fund we need.

问题是我们从哪获得资金。

His care is not how he will do it, but how well he will do it. → His care is not how to do it, but how well to do it.

他关心的不是怎么做，而是怎么做好它。

注意：在第2、第3点中，"疑问词＋不定式"的动作的执行者可根据上下文来确定。但不是所有的名词性从句都适用"疑问词＋不定式"来简化，否则会影响句意的准确性和完整性。

Exercises

I. Rewrite the following sentences using "interrogative + infinitive".

1. The old man didn't remember how many times a day he would take the medicine.
   _____

2. When we will stop using the medicine requires advice from a doctor.
   _____

3. Do you ask the doctor about who is to do the operation on you?
   _____

4. We are discussing whether we will invite him to join us in business or not.
   _____

5. The question is when we should withdraw our investment fund.
   _____

II. Make a choice from the four choices marked A, B, C and D.

6. I'm going on a field trip but I haven't decided_____.

   A. what to do   B. to do what

   C. where to go   D. to go where

7. This physics problem is too difficult. Can you show me _____?

    A. what to work it out   B. what to work out it

    C. how to work it out   D. how to work out it

8. There isn't any difference between the two. I really don't know _____.

    A. where to choose   B. which to choose

    C. to choose what   D. to choose which

9. The students do not know _____ this math problem.

    A. how to deal with   B. what to do

    C. how to do with   D. what to deal with

10. I have no idea when _____ her the bad news.

    A. will tell   B. telling   C. tell   D. to tell

III. Translate the following passage from Chinese into English and try to use at least one "interrogative + infinitive" in your translation.

    如果你是个慢性病患者，如高血压或糖尿病病人，你应该咨询医生服什么药、怎样服、服多少、饮食和生活习惯上注意什么等等。在你选择同时服用其他非处方药，比如，止痛药或退烧药时，除了仔细阅读说明书外，还要避免新药和原来的药因含有同样有效成分而产生过量危险，或相互产生反应。

    参考词汇：

    高血压 hypertension；糖尿病 diabetes；退烧药 antipyretic

_____

_____

_____

_____

_____

Have Some Fun

A woman and her husband approach their pharmacist, and begin to ask questions like if the pharmacy checks for medications past their expiration date and the reliability of a certain company that makes birth control pills. Finally, the pharmacist asks the couple what's the matter. The wife explains, "In spite of using birth control pills I continue to get pregnant." The pharmacist is astounded and asks the woman if she takes them every day. The woman replies, "My husband takes them every day." "What?" the pharmacist croaks. "Yep. After we read all those potential side-effects, my husband said 'Ah honey… I don't what you taking that stuff. It's too dangerous… let ME take them.' "

Unit 6 Drug Safety

Lead-in

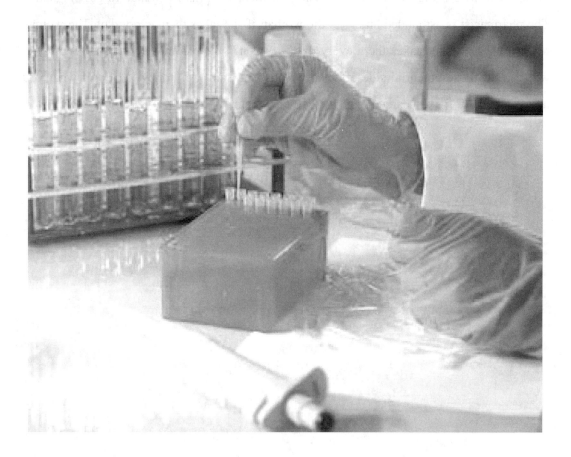

Food is the continuation of life; drug is the savior for health. However, in recent years, China's drug safety issues have become increasingly prominent, the major drug safety accidents occur from time to time, drug safety problem has been a serious threat to people's life and health.

Unit 6 Drug Safety

Speaking and Listening

Dialogue

At the Pharmacy (2)

Patient: Good morning. Can I have my prescription filled here?

Pharmacist: Yes, this is the hospital pharmacy. Would you please show me your prescription?

Patient: Okay. Here you are.

Pharmacist: Here is your medicine.

Patient: Could you please tell me how to take the medicine?

Pharmacist: This is spiramycin (螺旋霉素) tablet. Take two tablets each time, twice a day, better after meal.

Patient: How about this one? Is it also for internal use?

Pharmacist: No, it's only for gargling (含漱).

Patient: How should I take the painkiller?

Pharmacist: Take one tablet if you feel the pain, but no more than once every four hours.

Patient: How should I take these big balls?

Pharmacist: Chew and swallow the bits with water or you can also put them in water to melt them. Make sure to remove the wax before taking them.

Start New Dialogue

★ Discuss and role-play a conversation with your partner based on the given information.

You are a pharmacist in a pharmacy. A patient is asking you some questions about filling his or her prescription.

Stick Up Your Ears

★ Listen to the recording and fill in the blanks according to what you hear.

The State Council (国务院), China's Cabinet, recently issued a document on building a (1)_____ and specialized team of pharmaceutical drug inspectors (检验员). The document advances (2)_____ the pharmaceutical drug inspection system by establishing national and provincial teams of (3)_____ inspectors.

According to the document, the inspectors, who will be specialized professional personnel (4)_____ by the drug administration authorities, will conduct compliance confirmation and (5)_____ analysis inspections of medical drug research and production, including cosmetics, and medical (6)_____, to ensure they are developed and produced according to the law.

They will be an important force for (7)_____ drug supervision and ensuring drug safety.

The State Council medicine administration department and provincial level medicine administration departments are (8)_____ to have established a professional, specialized drug inspection system with (9)_____ inspectors as the main body and part-time inspectors as the supplement (10)_____ the next three years.

Reading and Writing

In-depth Reading

Drug Safety

Hong Kong has seen three serious drug-related incidents involving local pharmaceutical companies over just a month. It shows the good manufacturing practices (GMP) system has failed.

There are problems with all aspects of the pharmaceutical industry—production, sale and registration. Citizens are no longer confident

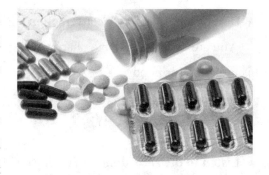

that medicines are safe. The first thing the Department of Health must do is to take such actions that citizens who need to take drugs will do so without worry. The government must carry out a comprehensive review of the drug safety system and reform it with a view to ending the pharmaceutical safety crisis and restoring confidence in Hong Kong's accreditation systems.

What has happened shows the drug incidents should not be regarded as isolated cases. Some problems are universal with local pharmaceutical companies. Apparently, that has everything to do with Hong Kong's imperfect drug safety system and the Department of Health's lax supervision.

Under the present system, pharmaceutical companies that meet the GMP standards are licensed by the Department of Health to sell their products in the territory. The department does not normally test their drugs. Its inspectors visit drug-makers once or twice a year to make sure that they meet all the requirements.

However, the department relies mainly on their reports to determine whether they have followed all the steps of process.

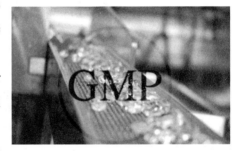

Whether GMP succeeds depends very much on pharmaceutical companies' self-discipline. However, what has happened shows there are so many loopholes in the system that it does not ensure drug safety. Relying on paperwork for monitoring drug-makers, the Department of Health cannot possibly detect problems. Furthermore, it has only 28 pharmacists. They monitor 25 pharmaceutical companies, 500 community pharmacies and 5,000 clinics. They also deal with the registration of traditional Chinese medicine. The strength of the department is out of all proportion to its workload.

Citizens' health is therefore exposed to huge risk. The government must learn a lesson from the bitter incidents and resolve to reform the drug safety system thoroughly.

It should be the government's long-term aim to find ways to further improve Hong Kong's accreditation systems. However, what it should do now is to restore confidence in drug safety. We may not pin high hopes on the Department of Health, which lacks staff. The only way of ending the confidence crisis is to require pharmaceutical companies to have their products tested by qualified third-party laboratories and submit their reports to the Department of Health for its perusal. The whole process must be sufficiently transparent so that citizens will know whether certain drugs are safe.

(426 words)

New Words & Expressions

pharmaceutical /ˌfɑːməˈsuːtɪkl/	adj.	制药（学）的
registration /ˌredʒɪˈstreʃn/	n.	登记；注册；挂号
accreditation /əˌkredɪˈteɪʃn/	n.	鉴定合格；达到标准
isolated /ˈaɪsəleɪtɪd/	adj.	偏远的；孤立的，单独的；孤独的；绝缘的
universal /ˌjuːnɪˈvɜːsl/	adj.	普遍的；通用的；全体的
apparently /əˈpærəntlɪ/	adv.	显然地；似乎，表面上
lax /læks/	adj.	不严格的，松懈的
supervision /ˌsuːpəˈvɪʒn/	n.	监督，管理
territory /ˈterətrɪ/	n.	领土，领域；范围，地域；版图
inspector /ɪnˈspektə(r)/	n.	检查员；巡视员
self-discipline /ˌselfˈdɪsəplɪn/	n.	自律；自我修养
loophole /ˈluːphəʊl/	n.	（法律、合同等的）漏洞，空子
workload /ˈwɜːkləʊd/	n.	工作量
thoroughly /ˈθʌrəlɪ/	adv.	彻底地，完全地
restore /rɪˈstɔː(r)/	vt.	恢复；修复；归还
pin /pɪn/	vt.	钉住；压住；将……用针别住
	n.	大头针，别针，针
submit /səbˈmɪt/	vt.	呈递；提交
perusal /pəˈruːzl/	n.	阅读；精读
transparent /trænsˈpærənt/	adj.	透明的；显然的

Notes to the Text

1. **GMP (good manufacturing practices)**：即生产质量管理规范，GMP 是一套适用于制药、食品等行业的强制性标准。简要地说，GMP 要求制药、食品等生产企业具备良好的生产设备、合理的生产过程、完善的质量管理和严格的检测系统，确保最终产品质量（包括食品安全卫生）符合法规要求。

2. Hong Kong has seen three serious drug-related incidents involving local pharmaceutical companies over just a month.

解析：involving local pharmaceutical companies over just a month 为现在分词引导的后置定语从句，相当于 which involve local pharmaceutical...。

译文：仅一个月，香港就发生了三起涉及本地制药公司的严重药物事件。

3. The first thing the Department of Health must do is to take such actions that citizens who need to take drugs will do so without worry.

解析：句子主干为：The first thing is to take such actions；the Department of Health must do 是定语从句，修饰 the first thing；citizens who need to take drugs will do so without worry 本身是一个包含定语从句的复合句，这个复合句又作定语从句修饰 such actions。

译文：卫生署必须做的第一件事是采取行动，让需要服用药物的公民服药时不再担心药物的安全性。

4. The government must carry out a comprehensive review of the drug safety system and reform it with a view to ending the pharmaceutical safety crisis and restoring confidence in Hong Kong's accreditation systems.

解析：carry out 表示"执行，实施"。

译文：政府必须全面检讨药物安全制度，并进行改革，以结束药物安全危机，恢复市民对香港药物认证系统的信心。

5. The only way of ending the confidence crisis is to require pharmaceutical companies to have their products tested by qualified third-party laboratories and submit their reports to the Department of Health for its perusal.

解析：have their products tested 源于短语 have sth. done，意为"某事由……做"，文中指"由……检测产品"；submit their reports to 源于动词短语 submit...to...，意为"向……提交"。

译文：结束信任危机的唯一方法是要求制药公司让合格的第三方实验室对其产品进行检测，并向卫生署提交报告供其审阅。

药学英语

Post-reading Tasks

I. Answer the following questions according to the text.

1. What is the first thing the Department of Health must do?
   _____

2. Under the present system, how the Department of Health works?
   _____

3. Does the Department of Health test the drugs?
   _____

4. GMP's success depends very much on pharmaceutical companies' self-discipline, why does it work inefficiently?
   _____

5. What's the only way to end the confidence crisis?
   _____

II. Complete the following statements with the words given below. Change the form if necessary.

accreditation	pin	collapse	pharmacist	inspector
isolate	apparently	restore	thoroughly	submit

6. The Premier _____ Mr. Bush as his representative.

7. When I arrived in Jerusalem, I spent three days there to _____ how the wall of Jerusalem looked like.

8. You can get some pills at the _____ across the street.

9. Despite their efforts the project _____.

10. When something goes wrong, we look for someone to _____ it on.

11. The balloon had landed in an _____ area.

12. The work has not been done very _____.

13. Your project must be _____ to the board by March 10.

14. I thought she had retired, but _____ she hasn't.

15. His job is _____ old paintings.

III. Read the following passage carefully and choose the best answer.

Your sensory and motor nerve cells can sometimes work together without involving your brain. What do you do if someone behind you suddenly makes a loud noise? What happens when a strong light is accidentally flashed in your eyes? The reaction to each of these events is a reflex. You do not have to think about a reflex. It happens automatically.

Reflexes are protective actions. Reflexes are very fast because the impulses are not carried as far as they are in a regular response reaction. In a reflex action, the impulse travels from a sensory receptor through a sensory nerve cell to the spinal cord. Association nerve cells in the spinal cord send the impulse directly to a motor nerve cell that carries out the response immediately.

Usually, a reflex begins when a sensory receptor is suddenly stimulated a great deal. Imagine that you are cooking at a hot stove and you accidentally steam your hand. The sensory receptors in your skin detect the change in temperature. Impulses begin in some of the sensory nerve cells in your hand and travel to your spinal cord. Then, the impulses pass from the spinal cord to motor nerve cells in your arm. Your arm muscles contract and pull your hand away from the stove. By this time, impulses traveling up your spinal cord have reached your brain. Your brain interprets what has just happened and gives you the message: "Hot." Luckily for you, your hand is already out of danger.

Reflexes help the body react quickly to changes in the environment. When impulses in a reflex travel just to your spinal cord, your body responds immediately in a regular response reaction, the impulse travels to the brain, slowing the response. If after the impulse arrives at the brain, you have to think about what to do, your response will take even longer.

16. This passage mainly talks about_____.
    A. what a reflex is   B. when a reflex will happens
    C. how a reflex happens   D. why a reflex happens

17. What major organ of the central nervous system is not involved in a reflex?
    A. The brain.   B. The spinal cord.

C. The sensory receptor.   D. The sensory and motor nerve cells.

18. Which of the following will not result in a person's reflex?

    A. Making a loud sudden noise.   B. Flashing a strong light in the darkness.

    C. Changing a traffic light.   D. Touching a hot frying-pan.

19. Which of the following is the last step of a reflex?

    A. From a sensory receptor to a sensory nerve cell.

    B. From a sensory nerve cell to the spinal cord.

    C. From the spinal cord to a motor nerve cell.

    D. From a motor nerve cell to the brain.

Practical Writing

GMP Certificate

Read and Understand

CERTIFICATE OF GOOD MANUFACTURING FOR

PHARMACEUTICAL PRODUCTS PEOPLE'S REPUBLIC OF CHINA

Certificate No.: M08**

Manufacturer: Zhejiang Jiangbei Pharmaceutical Co. Ltd.

Address: Zhang'an Street, Dongdai, Jiaojiang District, Taizhou City

Scope of Inspection: Active Pharmaceutical Ingredient (Simvastatin)

This is to certify that above-mentioned manufacturer compiles with the requirements of Chinese Good Manufacturing Practices for Pharmaceutical Products.

This certificate remains valid until 12/31/2015.

Issued By Zhejiang Food and Drug Administration

Date for Issuing 01/28/2011

CHINA FOOD AND DRUG ADMINISTRATION

GMP 是为保证药品在规定的质量下持续生产的体系。它是为把药品生产过程中的不合格的危险降低到最小而订立的。GMP 包含方方面面的要求，包括原料、人员、设施设备、生产过程、包装运输、质量控制等。"GMP"是英文 Good Manufacturing Practice 的缩写，中文的意思是"良好作业规范"或"优良制造标准"，是一种特别注重在生产过程中实施对产品质量与卫生安全的自主性 管理制度。它是一套适用于制药、食品等行业的强制性标准。

《药品 GMP 证书》有效期一般为 5 年。新开办药品生产企业的《药品 GMP 证书》有效期为 1 年。药品生产企业应在有效期届满前 6 个月，重新申请药品 GMP 认证。新开办药品生产企业《药品 GMP 证书》有效期届满前 3 个月申请复查，复查合格后，颁发有效期为 5 年的《药品 GMP 证书》。

Useful Information

证书编号：Certificate No.
企业名称：
企业地址：英文地址的书写是从小到大的顺序，按门牌号、街道名、城市名、国家名的顺序依次书写
认证的范围：Scope of Approval
颁发日期：Date of Issuing
有效日期：valid until

Writing Practice

Complete the GMP Certificate based on the given information.

无锡福祈制药有限公司（Wuxi Fortune Pharmaceutical Co., Ltd.）原料药 [(螺旋霉素 (Spiramycin)、利福喷丁 (Rifapentine)]、硬胶囊剂、片剂符合《药品生产质量管理规范》要求，于 2018 年 6 月 15 日通过江苏省食品药品监督管理局 GMP 认证。公司地址为无锡市荣洋一路 2 号。

CERTIFICATE OF GOOD MANUFACTURING PRACTICES FOR
PHARMACEUTICAL PRODUCTS PEOPLE'S REPUBLIC OF CHINA

Certificate No.: JS2018****

Manufacturer: _____

Address: _____

Scope of Inspection: _____

This is to certify that above mentioned manufacturer compiles with the requirements of Chinese Good Manufacturing Practices for Pharmaceutical Products.

This certificate remains valid until _____

Issued By _____

Date for Issuing _____

CHINA FOOD AND DRUG ADMINISTRATION

Grammar

Post-positive Attributive
后置定语

我们已经学习了定语从句作后置定语、现在分词作后置定语以及过去分词作后置定语，本单元将介绍剩下的几种定语后置的类型。

非谓语动词有三种形式：现在分词、过去分词和动词不定式，它们都可以作后置定语。现在分词和过去分词作后置定语的情况我们已经讨论过，下面我们来介绍动词不定式作后置定语、介词短语作后置定语、形容词作后置定语和单个词作后置定语。

1. 动词不定式作后置定语

（1）动词不定式与所修饰词之间是主谓关系，被修饰词为逻辑主语。

He is always the first to come.

他总是第一个来。

Are you going to the meeting to be held tomorrow?

你打算去参加明天举行的会议吗？

（2）动词不定式与所修饰词之间是动宾关系，被修饰词为直接宾语。

They are looking for a place to live.

他们正在寻找住处。

He had a big family to support.

他有一大家人要养活。

（3）动词不定式对所修饰词起阐释作用。

She had no chance to go school in those years.

那些年，她没机会上学。

We got no instruction to leave the city.

我们没有接到离开这个城市的指示。

2. 介词短语作后置定语

介词短语表明所修饰词的时间、地点、范围、类别、来源等。

The weather in Beijing is colder than that in Guangzhou.

北京的天气比广州冷。

His love for his country is very great.

他很热爱自己的国家。

3. 形容词短语作后置定语

Italian is a language very difficult to learn.

意大利语是一门非常难学的语言。

The leaders present at the meeting totaled eight.

出席会议的领导共有八人。

4. 单个词作后置定语

（1）英语中有些以 a 为词首的形容词，如 alone，alike，aware，ashamed 等。

The girl asleep soundly is my younger sister.

正在熟睡的小女孩是我的妹妹。

He is the greatest writer alive.

他是当代最伟大的作家。

（2）以后缀 -able，-ible 结尾的形容词。

I know the actor suitable for the part.

我认识适合扮演这个角色的演员。

Are there any tickets available?

还有票吗？

（3）所修饰词是不定代词时。

There is something important in today's newspaper.

今天的报纸上有条重要新闻。

He wanted to get someone reliable to help in this work.

他想找个可靠的人帮忙做这项工作。

Exercises

I. Read the following statements carefully, and tick the ones including post-positive attributives.

☐ 1. The student who answers the question was John.

☐ 2. The weather in Beijing is colder than that in Guangzhou.

☐ 3. The girl asleep soundly is my young sister.

☐ 4. They built a highway leading into the mountains.

☐ 5. Italian is a language very difficult to learn.

II. Fill in each blank with the proper form of the word given in brackets.

6. The letter _____ (write) is to my father.

7. The matter _____ (discuss) is important.

8. I usually have a lot of meetings _____ (attend).

9. This is a difficult problem _____ (solve).

10. Everything _____ (use) in the house was taken away by him by force.

11. He is the only person _____ (rely).

12. During the winter, I like my house warm and _____ (comfort).

13. He was the only Englishman _____ (presence).

III. Translate a passage from Chinese into English and try to use at least one post-positive attributive in your translation.

在美国所有的新药必须要得到联邦食品与药品监督管理局的批准才能上市。所有药物都会有潜在的不良反应，所以，只有当某种药物的益处大于其风险时，它才有可能被批准上市。但是，对新药审批的检查需要很长时间，因此联邦食品与药品管理局在 1987 年出台一项规定，允许一些有价值的处于审批中的药物用于危重病人。

参考词汇：

批准上市 be approved to go to the market；危重病人 critically ill patients

Have Some Fun

A light heart lives long. —William Shakespeare
豁达者长寿。——威廉·莎士比亚
Sloth, like rust, consumes faster than labor wears. —Benjamin Franklin
懒惰像生锈一样，比操劳更能消耗身体。——本杰明·富兰克林
Cheerfulness is the best promoter of health. —Thomas Alva Addison
快乐最利于健康。——托马斯·阿尔瓦·爱迪生

Unit 7 Drug Development

Lead-in

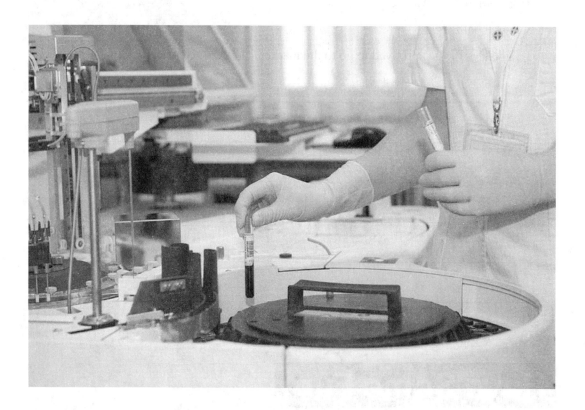

Drug development is the process of bringing a new pharmaceutical drug to the market once a lead compound has been identified through the process of drug discovery. It includes pre-clinical research and clinical trials and may include the step of obtaining regulatory approval to market the drug. Have you ever known anything about drug development? Do you know anyone who contributed to the development of new drugs?

Speaking and Listening

Dialogue

At the Pharmacy (3)

Patient: Excuse me. I need to refill this prescription.

Pharmacist: It says on the bottle here that you can have two refills.

Patient: Yes, I need to refill it today.

Pharmacist: Alright. I'm sorry, Miss. According to our file, this prescription has already been refilled twice.

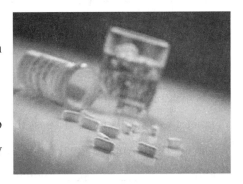

Patient: I was worried about that. I couldn't remember if I had it refilled twice yet or not.

Pharmacist: Well, it looks like you have. You will need to see your doctor to get a new prescription.

Patient: Listen. This is an emergency. I tried to call my doctor, but he is out of town. So I can't see him in time. I need this medicine. It is for skin condition. I've run out. Can you just refill it once more?

Pharmacist: I'm sorry, Miss. I can't do it. I understand your problem. But it is against the law for us to sell certain medicines without a prescription. I can't do anything about it. Sorry.

Start New Dialogue

★ Discuss and role-play a conversation with your partner based on the given information.

Imagine you are a pharmacist. A patient is asking you to refill his prescription.

Stick Up Your Ears

★ Listen to the recording and fill in the blanks according to what you hear.

Scientists have developed a new cancer drug. So far, they have tested it only in laboratory animals. The drug is (1) _____ to enter and kill cancer cells, but not healthy cells. First, the drug enters the cancer cells and stops their (2) _____ of blood. Then it (3) _____ poison to destroy the cancer cells. Researchers at the Massachusetts Institute of Technology (MIT, 麻省理工学院) in Cambridge (4) _____ the study. The results appeared in *Nature* magazine. A school report called the drug an "anticancer smart bomb".

Ram Sasisekharan is a professor at MIT. He says that his team had to solve three problems. They had to find a way to destroy the blood vessels, then to (5) _____ the growth of new ones. But they also needed the blood vessels to supply chemicals to destroy the cancer. So, the researchers designed a two-part "nanocell" (纳米细胞). The cell is measured in nanometers (纳米), or one thousand millionth of a meter. The scientists say that it was small enough to pass through the blood (6) _____ of the cancer, but it was too big to enter normal blood vessels. The surface of the nanocells also helped them to avoid (7) _____ defenses. The scientists designed the cell as a balloon inside a balloon. They filled the outer part with a drug that caused the blood vessels to die. That (8) _____ the blood supply and put the nanocells inside the cancer. Then, the nanocells slowly released drugs to kill the cancer cells. The team says that the (9) _____ killed the cancer and avoided healthy cells (10) _____ than other treatments.

Reading and Writing

In-depth Reading

The Drug Development Process

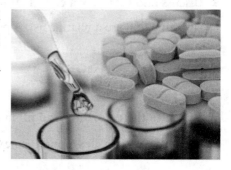

The process of drug development can be divided into five steps: discovery and development, preclinical research, clinical research, FDA review and FDA post-market safety monitoring.

Step 1: Discovery and Development

Typically, researchers discover new drugs for over

2 years through new insights into a disease process, many tests of molecular compounds, existing treatments, or new technologies. At this stage in the process, thousands of compounds may be potential candidates for development as a medical treatment. After early testing, however, only a small number of compounds look promising and call for further study.

Step 2: Preclinical Research

Before testing a drug in people, researchers must find out whether it has the potential to cause serious harm, also called toxicity. Usually, the researchers have to spend 2 to 5 years on preclinical studies, which must provide detailed information on dosing and toxicity levels. After preclinical testing, researchers review their findings and decide whether the drug should be tested in people.

Step 3: Clinical Research

Clinical research refers to studies, or trials, that are done in people. As the developers design the clinical study, they will consider what they want to accomplish for each of the different Clinical Research Phases and begin the Investigational New Drug Process (IND), a process they must go through before clinical research begins.

Clinical Research Phase Studies

Phase	Study Participants	Length of Study	Purpose
Phase 1	20 to 100 healthy volunteers or people with the disease/condition	Several months	Safety and dosage
Phase 2	Up to several hundred people with the disease/condition	Several months to 2 years	Efficacy and side effects
Phase 3	300 to 3,000 volunteers who have the disease or condition	1 to 4 years	Efficacy and monitoring of adverse reactions
Phase 4	Several thousand volunteers who have the disease or condition		Safety and efficiancy

Step 4: FDA Review

If a drug developer has evidence from its early tests and preclinical and clinical research that a drug is safe and effective for its intended use, the company can file an application to market the drug. Examining thoroughly all submitted data on the drug, the FDA review team

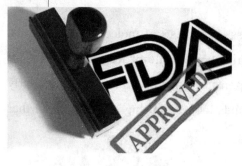

makes a decision to approve or not to approve it. Often, though, remaining issues need to be resolved before the drug can be approved for marketing, and the NDA contains sufficient data for FDA to determine the safety and effectiveness of a drug.

Step 5: FDA Post-market Safety Monitoring

The true picture of a product's safety actually evolves over the months and even years that make up a product's lifetime in the marketplace. FDA reviews reports of problems with prescription and over-the-counter drugs, and can decide to add cautions to the dosage or usage information, as well as other measures for more serious issues.

To conclude, it takes 10 to 20 years to develop a new drug. And the process is rather complicated.

(473 words)

New Words & Expressions

preclinical /priːˈklɪnɪk(ə)l/	adj.	临床前的，潜伏期的；临床使用前的
clinical /ˈklɪnɪkl/	adj.	临床的；诊所的
insight /ˈɪnsaɪt/	n.	洞察力，深入了解
molecular /məˈlekjələ(r)/	adj.	分子的，由分子组成的
candidate /ˈkændɪdət/	n.	候选人，候补人
toxicity /tɒkˈsɪsətɪ/	n.	毒性，毒力
trial /ˈtraɪəl/	n.	试验；审讯
accomplish /əˈkʌmplɪʃ/	vt.	完成；实现；达到
efficacy /ˈefɪkəsɪ/	n.	功效，效力
evolve /ɪˈvɒlv/	vt.	发展，进化
complicated /ˈkɒmplɪkeɪtɪd/	adj.	难懂的，复杂的
call for		要求；需要
clinical research phase		临床研究阶段
make up		组成；补足
to conclude		最后；总而言之

Notes to the Text

1. The process of drug development can be divided into five steps: discovery and development, preclinical research, clinical research, FDA review and FDA post-market safety monitoring.

解析：can be divided into 为含有情态动词的被动语态。

译文：药品研发的过程分五个阶段：发现与开发阶段、临床前试验阶段、临床试验阶段、食品药品监督管理局审查阶段和食品药品监督管理局上市后安全监测阶段。

2. Usually, the researchers have to spend 2 to 5 years on preclinical studies, which must provide detailed information on dosing and toxicity levels.

解析：spend (time) on … 指 "花费（时间）在……上"；which must provide… 为非限制性定语从句，修饰限定 preclinical studies。

译文：通常，研究人员需要花费 2 到 5 年的时间进行临床前研究，这些研究必须提供有关剂量和毒性水平的详细信息。

3. Often, though, remaining issues need to be resolved before the drug can be approved for marketing, and the NDA contains sufficient data for FDA to determine the safety and effectiveness of a drug.

解析：though 表示转折 "然而"；NDA 为 New Drug Application 的缩写。

译文：然而，往往在药物被批准上市之前，剩下的问题需要得到解决，新药申请中也要包含足够的数据供 FDA 来确定药物的安全性和有效性。

4. If a drug developer has evidence from its early tests and preclinical and clinical research that a drug is safe and effective for its intended use, the company can file an application to market the drug.

解析：if 引导条件状语从句；is safe and effective for 表示转折 "然而"。

译文：如果药品研发企业从药品早期试验、临床前试验及临床研究中获得证据，证明该药对其预期用途是安全有效的，则该企业可以提出申请将该药推向市场。

药学英语

Post-reading Tasks

I. Answer the following questions according to the text.

1. How many steps can the process of drug development be divided into? What are they?
   _____

2. What should researchers find out before testing a drug in people?
   _____

3. What is the process researchers must go through before clinical research begins?
   _____

4. On what condition could a company file an application to market a drug?
   _____

5. How does the FDA carry out post-market safety monitoring?
   _____

II. Complete the following statements with the words or phrase given below. Change the form if necessary.

insight	candidate	promising	absorb	distribute
accomplish	go through	evolve	complicated	submit

6. There were a large number of _____ for the job.

7. Last year, our company _____ a bad time.

8. The research produced _____ results.

9. If we'd all work together, I think we could _____ our goal.

10. Applying that technology on a larger scale turned out to be more _____.

11. I hope you have gained some _____ into the difficulties we face.

12. Let the rice cook until it _____ all the water.

13. If you want to apply for the job, you need to fill in and _____ an application form.

14. They agreed that a fair _____ of income and wealth is necessary.

15. In the course of _____, some birds have lost the power of flight.

III. Read the following passage carefully and choose the best answer.

Doctors may now be able to stop many heart attacks. An important new study reports that doctors have a new drug. This drug is called TPA. It may be better than any other heart drugs.

Many doctors now use a drug called streptokinase (链激酶). But this drug sometimes causes problems for patients. It can even cause bleeding in the brain. Some doctors do not use streptokinase. Streptokinase can save about 1/3 of the people with heart attacks. But TPA will save about 2/3.

One reason TPA can help more people is because of time. This new drug is easier and faster to use. It will give doctors more time in hospitals. Then they can study the problem well. People with heart problems can also keep some TPA at home. When a heart attack starts, they can take some TPA right away. Then they will have time to get to the hospital. This is important because about 860,000 people in the United States die before they get to the hospital.

This is another reason why TPA is good news for people with heart attacks. According to the study, it is much safer; it doesn't cause other problems like streptokinase does. TPA works only on the heart. It does not have an effect on the blood or cause bleeding.

Doctors plan to do more studies about TPA. They need to test this new drug on many more people with heart attacks. But in a few years, many doctors and hospitals will probably start using this exciting new drug.

16. In your opinion, the best title for this passage is _____.

    A. Heart Attacks

    B. A New Drug for Heart Attacks

    C. The Cause of Heart Attacks

    D. A Drug Called Streptokinase

17. The story says that TPA _____.

    A. is safer and faster than the old drug

    B. is very dangerous

    C. is slower and harder to use than the old drug

    D. causes many problems

18. This new drug may mean _____.

   A. more people will die from heart attacks

   B. the same number of people will die from heart attacks

   C. fewer people will die from heart attacks

   D. no one will die from heart attacks

19. Which of the following is TRUE?

   A. Streptokinase is the new drug for heart attacks.

   B. TPA can save fewer people with heart attacks than streptokinase.

   C. People who take TPA at home before they go to hospital must be very careful.

   D. Probably TPA will be widely used in the following years.

Practical Writing

IND Application Form

Useful Information

> The IND (Investigational New Drug) application form (新药临床试验申请表) mainly consists of the following parts:
>
> (1) Name of Sponsor 申请人姓名
>
> (2) Date of Submission 提交日期
>
> (3) Sponsor Address 申请人地址
>
> (4) Telephone Number 电话号码
>
> (5) Name(s) of Drug 药品名称
>
> (6) IND Number (If previously assigned) 新药申请编号
>
> (7) (Proposed) Indication for Use 使用说明
>
> (8) Phase(s) of Clinical Investigation to be conducted 临床调查阶段
>
> (9) Name and Title of the person responsible for monitoring the conduct and progress of the clinical investigations 临床调查负责人的姓名和职称
>
> (10) Name(s) and title(s) of the person(s) responsible for review and evaluation of information relevant to the safety of the drug 药品安全评估负责人的姓名和职称

Writing Practice

Complete the IND application form in English based on the information given in Chinese.

双环醇片（Bicyclol），商品名"百赛诺"，由中国医学科学院、中国协和医科大学药物开发，是我国第一个具有自主知识产权一类抗肝炎合成创新药物。1996年12月经卫生部批准进入临床试验，2001年9月获得原SDA颁发的新药证书及生产批准文，由北京协和药厂生产上市。目前已在全球16个国家和地区获得20年发明专利保护，在国内享有12年的行政保护期。

现由中国医学科学院药物研究所著名药物化学家李志强教授向美国FDA申请新药。提交日期：2016年5月8日；地址：中国北京市东城区东直门内南小街16号；邮编：100700；联系电话：(86)010-64018811。中国中医科学院王晓波教授负责临床调查工作，由中国中医科学院魏正清教授和刘霖教授负责药品安全评估。

DEPARTMENT OF HEALTH AND HUMANSEVICES Food and Drug Administration Investigational New Drug Application (IND) (Title 21, Code of Federal Regulations (CFR) Part 312)		
1. Name of Sponsor		
2. Date of Submission		
3. Sponsor Address	Address 1 (Street address, P.O. box, company name c/o)	
	Address 2 (Apartment, suite, unit, building, floor, etc.)	
	City	State/Province/Region
	Country	ZIP/Postal Code
4. Telephone Number (Include country codes if applicable and area code)		
5. Names of Drug (Include all available names: Trade, Generic, Chemical, or Code)		

6. IND Number (If previously assigned)	
7. (Proposed) Indication for Use	Is this indication for a rare disease (prevalence <200,000 in U.S.)? ☐ Yes ☐ No
	Does this product have an FDA Orphan Designation for this indication? ☐ Yes ☐ No | If yes, provide the Orphan Designation number for this indication:
8. Phase(s) of Clinical Investigation to be conducted	☐ Phase 1 ☐ Phase 2 ☐ Phase 3 ☐ Other (Specify): _____
9. Name and Title of the person responsible for monitoring the conduct and progress of the clinical investigations _____	
10. Name(s) and Title(s) of the person(s) responsible for review and evaluation of information relevant to the safety of the drug	

Grammar

Present Participle Used as Adverbial
现在分词作状语

现在分词（动词+ing）作状语，修饰动词，相当于状语从句，它表示的动作是主语动作的一部分。句子的主语必须是状语的逻辑主语，并且主语与作状语的分词之间呈逻辑上的主谓关系。

Seeing from the top of the hill, we can see our beautiful school.

从山顶望下去，我们就能看到我们美丽的学校。(seeing 和该句主语 we 之间存在

逻辑上的主谓关系，即 see 的动作是由句子主语 we 发出的)

现在分词作状语，可表示伴随、条件、时间、方式、让步、原因、结果等。

1. 现在分词作伴随状语

I gazed into the dark sky, thinking about where I would belong.

我凝望着漆黑的夜空，思索着路在何方。

2. 现在分词作条件状语

Speaking in English every day, you will master this language step by step.

每天都用英语说话，你会一步一步掌握这门语言。

(相当于 if 引导的条件状语从句：If you speak in English everyday, you will…)

3. 现在分词作时间状语

Seeing the actors singing and dancing, the little baby did likewise.

当看到演员们载歌载舞的时候，小宝宝也学着手舞足蹈。

(相当于 when 引导的时间状语从句 when he saw the actors singing and dancing, the little baby…)

4. 现在分词作让步状语

Being a kid, he has much knowledge about love affairs.

虽然是个孩子，他知道很多关于爱情的事。

(相当于 though 引导的让步状语从句：Though he is a kid, he…)

5. 现在分词作原因状语

Not having prepared well, the speaker paused at times.

由于之前没有准备好，这个发言人老是停顿。

(相当于 because 引导的原因状语从句：Because he had not prepared well, the speaker…)

6. 现在分词作结果状语

He dropped a cup onto the floor, breaking it into pieces.

他将杯子掉在地上，摔碎了。

(相当于结果状语从句：He dropped a cup onto the floor so that the cup was broken into pieces.)

注意：如分词表示的动作不是句中主语发出或承受的，即为误用。

Exercises

I. There are two English versions for each of the following Chinese sentences. Judge which one is correctly written referring to the use of present participle as adverbials.

1. 从窗户看出去，我们看见一个漂亮的花园。

   a. Looking out through the window, the garden was beautiful.

   b. Looking out through the window, we saw a beautiful garden.

2. 我看着晚报的时候，一只狗开始叫起来。

   a. Reading the evening newspaper, a dog started barking.

   b. I was reading the evening newspaper when a dog started barking.

3. 听到这个消息，她忍不住哭了。

   a. Hearing the news, she cried out sadly.

   b. Hearing the news, tears ran down her face.

4. 如果你努力学习，你的梦想就一定会实现。

   a. Working hard with a strong will, your dream will certainly come true.

   b. Working hard with a strong will, you'll certainly make your dream come true.

II. Please rewrite the following sentences using present participle phrases as adverbials.

5. When she opened the window, she saw a butterfly flying into the room.
   _____

6. As he was ill, he didn't attend the wedding ceremony of his best friend.
   _____

7. If you work hard, you will succeed sooner or later.
   _____

8. Although they knew it was not fair, they made me pay for the damage.
   _____

9. He lay on the grass, and stared at the sky for a long time.
   _____

Unit 7 Drug Development

III. Translate a passage from Chinese into English and try to use at least one present participle phrase as adverbial in your translation.

作为一种古老的疾病，人类对疟疾的记载已经有 4000 多年历史。疟疾的传播非常广泛，中国古代称之为"瘴气"，意大利语中疟疾的意思是"坏空气"，表明中西方对这种疾病有大体相同的认识。人类对付疟疾的药物分别来源于两种植物——金鸡纳树和青蒿。2015 年 10 月，中国女药学家屠呦呦因发现青蒿素，与来自其他国家的另外两位科学家共享 2015 年度诺贝尔生理学或医学奖。

参考词汇：

疟疾 malaria；瘴气 miasma；金鸡纳树 cinchona；

青蒿 Artemisia apiacea 或 sweet wormwood；青蒿素 artemisinin；

2015 年度诺贝尔生理学或医学奖 2015 Nobel Prize in Physiology or Medicine

_____

_____

_____

_____

_____

_____

Have Some Fun

Take a walk after meals. — Sun Simiao

饭毕当行走。——孙思邈

A bad diet kills a man soon. —Li Shizhen

饮食不节，杀人顷刻。——李时珍

The purpose of scientific research is not to fight for fame or fortune. — Tu Youyou

科学研究不是为了争名夺利。——屠呦呦

Unit 8 Pharmaceutical Sales and Marketing

Lead-in

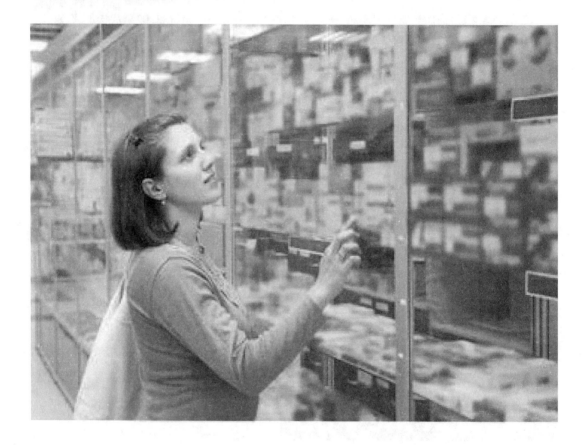

As a special kind of commodity, the marketing of drugs is also very special. So the manufacturers are very focused on the powerful marketing **strategy** as a competitive weapon. Do you know anything about pharmaceutical **sales** and marketing? In **this unit**, we will **talk** about the present **status** of the domestic and international **pharmaceutical sales and** marketing.

Speaking and Listening

Dialogue

Selling a Drug

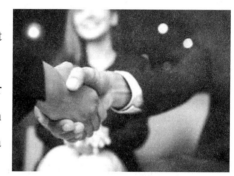

Andy: I'm glad that you can see me today.

Tan: Don't mention it, Andy. You are an important supplier to me.

Andy: Mr. Tan, the reason I'm here today is that our company has imported a new acne cream from the U.S. I wonder if you like to have a look?

Tan: Frankly speaking, the product you supplied to us before wasn't that effective. A lot of our customers have complained about it.

Andy: Mr. Tan, let me assure you one thing. This new product is really much better than the previous one. You have to try it to believe it.

Tan: Well, let me talk to my associates about this. I'll get back to you in a few days. In the mean time, just leave a sample here.

Andy: Thanks for your consideration.

Start New Dialogue

★ **Discuss and role-play a conversation with your partner based on the given information.**

Imagine you are a supplier of drugs. You want to sell a new kind of drugs to a big pharmacy. So you will have a conversation with a manager of this pharmacy.

Stick Up Your Ears

★ **Listen to the recording and fill in the blanks according to what you hear.**

Pharmaceutical sales jobs can involve intense studying and testing especially when launching a new pharmaceutical product. Pharmaceutical sales jobs (1)_____ the pharmaceutical sales representative to understand basic human anatomy (人体解剖学), physiology and (2)_____ pathology (病理学). In a pharmaceutical sales jobs you must also know the (3)_____, usage, and side effects of the pharmaceutical products your company represents (4) _____ now the competitor's pharmaceutical products in order to sell against them.

Often seen as a "dream job" or "piece of cake" position, most pharmaceutical sales (5) _____ will gladly debate this with anyone. A typical day for a pharmaceutical sales representative (6) _____ "calling on" or "detailing" 8~10 physicians a day and often 3~5 pharmacists a day. Many pharmaceutical sales representatives do this while covering a territory ranging from a 60~200 mile radius. Most pharmaceutical sales representatives are (7) _____ for covering 100~200 physicians in their area.

Access to these physicians can be very difficult and often provide a (8)_____ to even the most senior pharmaceutical sales representative. Creativity is important to help the sales representative gain (9) _____ to difficult to see physicians. The typical sales call is often less than 90 seconds (10) _____ the sales representative's sales skills are perfected to grab the physician's attention.

Reading and Writing

In-depth Reading

Pfizer: One of the World's Largest Pharmaceutical Companies

Pfizer, Inc. is an American multinational pharmaceutical corporation headquartered in New York City, with its research headquarters in Groton, Connecticut. It is among the world's largest pharmaceutical companies by revenues.

Pfizer was founded by cousins Charles Pfizer

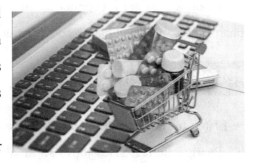

and Charles F. Erhart in New York City in 1849 as a manufacturer of fine chemicals. Pfizer's discovery of Terramycin (oxytetracycline) in 1950 put it on a path towards becoming a research-based pharmaceutical company. Pfizer is listed on the New York Stock Exchange, and its shares have been a component of the Dow Jones Industrial Average since April 2004.

Pfizer is organized into nine principal operating divisions: Primary Care, Specialty Care, Oncology, Emerging Markets, Established Products, Consumer Healthcare, Nutrition, Animal Health, and Capsugel. In May 2015, Pfizer and a Bar-Ilan University laboratory announced a partnership based on the development of medical DNA nanotechnology.

Pfizer's research and development activities are organized into two principal groups: the Pharma Therapeutics Research & Development Group, which focuses on the discovery of small molecules and related modalities; and the Bio Therapeutics Research & Development Group, which focuses on large-molecule research, including vaccines.

On September 1, 2011 Pfizer announced that it had agreed to a 10-year lease of more than 180,000 square feet of research space from MIT in a building to be constructed at 610 Main Street South, just north of the MIT campus in Cambridge, Massachusetts, U.S. The space would house Pfizer's Cardiovascular, Metabolic and Endocrine Disease Research Unit and its Neuroscience Research Unit — and Pfizer anticipates moving into the space once it was completed in late 2013.

Besides, Pfizer cares about its employees very much. Pfizer received a 100% rating on the Corporate Equality Index released by the Human Rights Campaign starting in 2004, the third year of the report. In 2007, Pfizer's Canadian division was named one of Canada's Top 100 Employers, as published in *Maclean's Magazine*, the only research-based pharmaceutical company to receive this honor.

Pfizer also concerns for the developing world health issues. Pfizer provides the antifungal drug fluconazole without charge to governmental and non-governmental organizations in developing countries with more than 1% HIV and AIDS prevalence. The company has also pledged to provide up to 480 million doses of its anti-pneumococcal vaccine at deeply discounted rates to children and infants in developing countries in collaboration with the GAVI Alliance. In 2012 Pfizer and the Gates Foundation announced a joint effort to provide 3 million women in the developing world with affordable access to Pfizer's long lasting injectable contraceptive, medroxyprogesterone acetate.

(420 words)

New Words & Expressions

multinational /ˌmʌltɪˈnæʃnəl/	adj.	跨国的；多国的
component / kəmˈpəʊnənt/	n.	成分；组分；零件；[数] 要素
nanotechnology /ˌnænəʊtekˈnɒlədʒɪ/	n.	纳米技术，毫微技术；纤技术
molecule /ˈmɒlɪkjuːl/	n.	分子；微小颗粒
therapeutics /ˌθerəˈpjuːtɪks/	n.	治疗学，疗法
anticipate /ænˈtɪsɪpeɪt/	v.	预见；预料；预感；先于……行动
antifungal /ˌæntɪˈfʌŋɡəl/	adj.	抗真菌的，杀真菌的
prevalence /ˈprevələns/	n.	流行；盛行；普遍；（疾病等的）流行程度
infant /ˈɪnfənt/	n.	婴儿，幼儿；未成年人；初学者，生手
medroxyprogesterone /meˌdrɒksɪprəʊˈdʒestərəʊn/	n.	甲孕酮，醋酸甲羟孕酮，安宫黄体酮
acetate /ˈæsɪteɪt/	n.	醋酸酯；醋酸盐；醋酸纤维；醋酸人造丝
in collaboration with		与……和合作
fine chemicals		精制化学药品
anti-pneumococcal vaccine		抗肺炎球菌疫苗
New York Stock Exchange		纽约证券交易所
Dow Jones Industrial Average		道琼斯工业平均指数
HIV (Human Immunodeficiency Virus)		艾滋病病毒
AIDS (Acquired Immune Deficiency Syndrome)		艾滋病，获得性免疫缺乏综合征
Gates Foundation		盖茨夫妇基金会
GAVI		全球疫苗免疫联盟

Unit 8 Pharmaceutical Sales and Marketing

Notes to the Text

1. Pfizer's research and development activities are organized into two principal groups: the Pharma Therapeutics Research & Development Group, which focuses on the discovery of small molecules and related modalities; and the Bio Therapeutics Research & Development Group, which focuses on large-molecule research, including vaccines.

解析：文中两个 which focuses on... 均为非限制性定语从句。

译文：辉瑞的研究和开发活动分为两个主要的小组：一个是药物治疗研究和开发小组，其主要工作是发现小分子及相关模式；另一个是生物疗法研发小组，该小组专注于包括疫苗在内的大分子研究。

2. On September 1, 2011 Pfizer announced that it had agreed to a 10-year lease of more than 180,000 square feet of research space from MIT in a building to be constructed at 610 Main Street South, just north of the MIT campus in Cambridge, Massachusetts, US.

解析：it had agreed... 为过去完成时；just north of the MIT campus in Cambridge, Massachusetts, US 为 610 Main Street South 的同位语。

译文：2011年9月1日，辉瑞公司宣布与麻省理工学院签订了一项为期10年的租赁合同，将租用麻省理工学院位于美国马萨诸塞州剑桥市的缅因南街610号的一幢大楼里超过18万平方英尺的地方用作研究。

3. The company has also pledged to provide up to 480 million doses of its anti-pneumococcal vaccine at deeply discounted rates to children and infants in developing countries in collaboration with the GAVI Alliance.

解析：at deeply discounted rates 意为"以极低的折扣"。

译文：该公司还承诺与全球疫苗和免疫联盟合作，以极低的价格向发展中国家的儿童和婴儿提供多达4.8亿剂抗肺炎球菌疫苗。

4. In 2012 Pfizer and the Gates Foundation announced a joint effort to provide 3 million women in the developing world with affordable access to Pfizer's long lasting injectable contraceptive, medroxyprogesterone acetate.

解析：access to 意为"有权使用；通向……的入口"。

译文：2012年，辉瑞公司和盖茨基金会宣布共同努力，为发展中国家的300万妇女提供辉瑞公司长效注射避孕药物醋酸甲羟孕酮。

Post-reading Tasks

I. Decide whether the following statements are true (T) or false (F) according to the text.

☐ 1. Research headquarters of Pfizer are located in New York City.

☐ 2. Pfizer was set up by Charles F. Erhart himself in New York City in 1849 as a manufacturer of fine chemicals.

☐ 3. This company's research and development activities are organised into three principal groups.

☐ 4. The employees of Pfizer are not satisfied with their company.

☐ 5. Pfizer pay attention to the health issues of developing countries as well.

II. Read and match the words and their meanings.

6. antifungal   a. a person or company that produces goods in large quantities

7. manufacturer   b. the money that an organization receives from its business

8. multinational   c. an abstract part of something

9. component   d. the quality of prevailing generally; being widespread

10. prevalence   e. people have enough money to buy something

11. revenue   f. any agent that destroys or prevents the growth of fungi

12. affordable   g. the smallest amount of a chemical substance which can exist by itself.

13. molecule   h. involving or operating in several nations or nationalities

III. Read the following passage carefully and complete the following sentences.

Some companies are successful at marketing their drugs all over the world without making any major changes to them. Others have different formulations, advertising, and packaging in each country, due to differences in customs and laws.

Unit 8 Pharmaceutical Sales and Marketing

In France, medicines should not only cure a disease, but also look fresh and interesting. For example, pink eye drops have been popular here, which would be unthinkable in Germany. There people expect medicine to look more "clinical".

The strength of medicine varies considerably depending on what health authorities allow. In Germany, health authorities prefer companies to sell drugs with only one active ingredient, rather than in combinations. They also prefer lower drug dosages as compared to those set by authorities in other places.

In Russia, people prefer to buy over-the-counter products, like cold remedies or cough syrup, from people in pharmacies wearing white lab coats. So, when foreign companies try to introduce drugs here, they are asked for good in-pharmacy training programmes because the staff will have to answer many questions before people are willing to buy such cures.

Quality is important all over the world, but in Japan people take it one step further. They will reject a whole shipment of drugs if they find the smallest scratch or imperfection in one single package, even if it makes no difference to the product at all.

US patients tend to self-medicate and buy drugs online. Unlike in many countries, you'll also find many cheerful bright colored ads in magazines, which promote anti-depressants and other prescription drugs in the U.S. Of course, the next page is always full of all the warnings, possible side effects and things to ask your doctor about.

14. Some companies have different formulations, advertising, and packaging in each country, because_____.

15. Different from French people, Germans prefer to more _____ medicine.

16. If foreign companies try to introduce drugs in Russia, they will be asked for_____.

17. If Japanese people find even the smallest imperfection in one single package, they are likely to _____.

Practical Writing

E-mails

Read and Understand

From: John@sohu.com
To: Green123@sina.com
Cc: Tom123@sohu.com
Bcc: David@sina.com
Subject: Letter for Order
Date: September 1st, 2015

Dear Mr. Green,

We have discussed your offer of 5% and accept it on the terms quoted. We are prepared to give your medicines a trial, provided you can guarantee delivery on or before the 20th of September. The enclosed order is given strictly on this condition. We reserve the right of refusal of delivery and/or cancellation of the order after this date.

Yours sincerely,

John

Useful Information

药品订货的电子邮件一般由以下七个部分组成：

◆ Address—地址

From: 写信人 e-mail 地址

To: 收信人 e-mail 地址

Cc: 抄送收信人 e-mail 地址（Cc = Carbon Copy）

Bcc: 密送收信人 e-mail 地址（Bcc = Blind Carbon Copy）

◆ Subject—主题

Unit 8 Pharmaceutical Sales and Marketing

主题 (Subject) 框的内容应简明地概括邮件的内容，短的可以是一个单词，长的可以是一个名词性短语，也可以是完整的句子，但长度一般不超过 35 个字母。

◆ Date—日期

◆ Salutation—称呼

◆ Body—正文

◆ Complimentary Close—礼貌结束语

表示礼貌、谦恭、祝愿等的短语（如 All the best, Best wishes 或者 Yours truly ），后跟逗号。

◆ Signature of the Writer—写信人姓名

Writing Practice

Write an e-mail according to the information given in Chinese.

日期：2019 年 12 月 9 日

正文：

(1) 你作为药品销售经理 Alice Duff 感谢对方 (Caroline White) 订购了你公司的药品；

(2) 所订购的药品已经发出，大概一周后到达；

(3) 收到药品后请回复；

(4) 希望能继续与对方合作。

From: Alice@sina.com

To: Caroline@sina.com

Subject: _____

Date: _____

_____

_____

_____

_____

_____

Grammar

Subject Clause
主语从句

复合句中作主语的从句叫主语从句。引导主语从句的词有从属连词、连接代词、连接副词。

从属连词：that，whether。

连接代词：who, whom, whose, which, whoever, what, whatever, whichever。

连接副词：where, how, why, when。

1. 连接词的选用

(1) 由 what 和 that 引导的主语从句。

what 和 that 都可引导主语从句。what 除起连接作用外，还在主语从句中充当某些成分 (主语、宾语或表语)。而 that 在主语从句中不充当任何成分，只起连接词的作用。

What he wants is a new bicycle.

他想要一辆新自行车。

(2) 由 whether 引导的主语从句。

含有"是否"意思的主语从句，连接词不能用 if, 只能用 whether。

Whether we will hold a party in the open air next week is uncertain.

下周我们是否在户外举办派对还不确定。

(3) 由其他连接代词和连接副词引导的主语从句。

who, which, when, where, why, how 等连接代词和连接副词既有疑问含义，又起连接作用，同时在从句中充当各种成分。

Who she is doesn't concern me.

我在不在乎她是谁。

Where I spend my summer holiday is no business of yours.

我在哪里过暑假与你无关。

Which car you will choose to buy makes no difference.

你买哪一辆车都没什么影响。

(4) 由 whatever 和 whoever 引导的主语从句。

whatever 和 whoever 可以引导主语从句，并在句中作主语、宾语、表语等，不含疑问意义。whatever 相当于 anything that; whoever 相当于 anyone who。

Whoever (Anyone who) wants to enter into this school must take the exam.

无论谁想要进入这所学校，都必须参加考试。

Whatever(Anything that) she did was right.

她做的任何事都是正确的。

2. 形式主语 it 构成的主语从句

(1) 由连词 that 引导的主语从句，在大多数情况下可以用形式主语 it 代替，即将 it 放在句首，而将主语从句放在句末，以避免句子头重脚轻。

It is a matter of common experience that bodies are lighter in water than they are in air.

物体在水中比在空气中轻，这是大家共有的经验。

(2) 由连接代词、连接副词和连词 whether 引起的主语从句常可用先行词 it 作主语，而把主语从句放到后面去。

How many people we are to invite is still a question. → It is still a question how many people we are to invite.

我们要邀请多少人还是一个问题。

When we arrive doesn't matter. → It doesn't matter when we arrive.

我们什么时间到并不重要。

Whether it will do us harm or good remains to be seen. → It remains to be seen whether it will do us harm or good.

这对我们有害还是有利还说不准。

(3) 常见用 it 作形式主语的复合句结构

① It is a fact (a pity/no wonder/a good idea/a shame…) that…

It's a pity that you didn't come to my birthday party.

你没有来参加我的生日派对真是太遗憾了。

② It is important (necessary/advisable/desirable/imperative/true/strange/possible…) that… 需要注意的是，这类主语从句中，谓语动词很多为"(should) +动词原形"，即要用虚拟语气。

It is necessary that several nurses (should) stay.

留几个护士在这儿是很有必要的。

It is imperative that everyone (should) learn from practice.

每个人都应该从实践中学习。

③ It is reported (well-known/hoped/thought/expected/said/believed/decided/suggested/

ordered…) that…

  It is said that many people was killed in the earthquake.

  据说很多人在这次地震中丧生了。

  ④ It seems(appears/doesn't matter/makes no difference…) that…

  It makes no difference whether he will attend the meeting or not.

  他是否会参加会议无关紧要。

3. 主语从句中的否定前移

当用 it 作形式主语，而将主语从句放在句尾时，主语从句中的否定词常要前移至主句中。

  It doesn't seem that they are from the same university.

  看上去他们并不是来自同一所大学。

Exercises

I. There are ten incomplete sentences here. You are required to complete each sentences by choosing the appropriate answer from the four choices marked A, B, C and D.

1. It never occurred to me＿＿＿＿ you could succeed in persuading him to change his mind.

  A. which   B. what   C. that   D. if

2. It's obvious to the students＿＿＿＿ they should get well prepared for their future.

  A. as   B. that   C. which   D. whether

3. ＿＿＿＿ makes mistakes must correct them.

  A. What   B. That   C. Whoever   D. Whatever

4. It is uncertain＿＿＿＿ side effect the medicine will bring about, although about two thousand patients have taken it.

  A. that   B. how   C. what   D. whether

5. ＿＿＿＿ is no reason for dismissing her.

  A. Because she was a few minutes late   B. Owing to a few minutes late

  C. The fact that she was a few minutes late   D. Being a few minutes late

6. _____ we go swimming every day _____ us a lot of good.
   A. If, do　　　B. That, do　　　C. If, does　　　D. That, does

7. _____ we can't get seems better than ____ we have.
   A. What, what　B. What, that　C. That, that　D. That, what

8. _____ we'll go camping tomorrow depends on the weather.
   A. If　　　　B. Whether　　　C. That　　　D. Where

9. _____ is going to do the job will be decided by the Party committee.
   A. That　　　B. Why　　　C. How　　　D. Who

10. _____ leaves the room last ought to turn off the lights.
    A. Anyone　　B. The person　　C. Whoever　　D. Who

II. Mark the correct sentence(s) with C (=Correct). Then make necessary corrections in all the other sentences.

11. Light travels faster than sound is common knowledge.

12. It was requested that everyone made a speech at the meeting.

13. That the professor said is of great importance.

14. Whether she is coming or not doesn't matter too much.

15. No matter who breaks the rule will be punished.

16. When and where the meeting will be held still remain a question.

17. Where will the trees be planted has not been decided.

18. That you will win the medal seems unlikely.

III. Translate the following sentences from Chinese into English by using the subject clauses.

惠氏公司是全球 500 强企业之一，也是全球最大的以研发为基础的制药和保健品公司之一。惠氏在研究、开发、制造和销售药品、疫苗、生物制品、营养品和非处方药品等方面处于全球领先地位。惠氏的产品改善了全球各地人们的生活质量。惠氏的主要业务部门有惠氏药物部、惠氏健康药物部和动物保健品部等。

参考词汇：

惠氏公司 Wyeth Nutrition；疫苗 vaccine；领先 pioneer

Have Some Fun

The first wealth is health. —Ralph Waldo Emerson, American thinker
健康是人生第一财富。——美国思想家 爱默生
A little pill may well cure a great ill.
小药也可治大病。
Mischief comes by the pound and goes away by the ounce.
病来如山倒，病去如抽丝。

Glossary

A

accreditation	*n.*	委派；信赖；鉴定合格	U6
accurate	*adj.*	精确的，准确的；正确无误的	U1
active ingredient		有效成分，活性成分	U5
administration	*n.*	管理；实行；（政府）行政机关	U5
affordable	*adj.*	付得起的	U1
agree on		与……达成一致	U4
ailment	*n.*	小病；不安	U4
allergic	*adj.*	过敏的；过敏症的	U5
amount	*n.*	量，数量；总额；	U3
	vi.	等于；等同，接近；合计，总共	U3
analyte	*n.*	（被）分析物；分解物	U3
anesthetic	*n.*	（使局部或全身失去知觉的）麻醉剂，麻醉药	U1
apparently	*adv.*	显然地；似乎，表面上	U6
application	*n.*	申请(表，书)；应用	U2
as late as		迟至……才，一直到	U2
Ayurvedic Medicine		印度式草药疗法（世界上最古老的医疗系统之一）	U4

B

be associated with		与……有关，涉及	U2
be responsible for		对……负有责任	U4
be thought to		被认为	U2
biochemical	*adj.*	生物化学的	U1
biological	*adj.*	生物学的；与生物学相关的；有血亲关系的	
	n.	[药]生物制品，生物制剂	U1
botanical	*adj.*	植物学的	

	n.	植物性药材	U4
breastfeed	*v.*	用母乳喂养，哺乳	U5

C

candidate	*n.*	候选人，候补人	U7
capsule	*n.*	胶囊	U5
charged	*adj.*	充满感情的；紧张的，可能引起激烈反应的	U1
consistent	*adj.*	一致的；连续的；不矛盾的	U5
consist of		由……组成；包括	U3
contain	*vt.*	包含；容纳；含有，包括	U5
contribute to		有助于；贡献	U2
cosmetic	*n.*	化妆品；美发油，发蜡	U1

D

detect	*vt.*	查明，发现；侦查	U3
determine	*v.*	决定；决心；确定；测定	U3
distinguish from		辨别；将……与……区别开	U3
distribution	*n.*	财产分配	U1
dozens of		几十；许多	U4
drug facts		药品说明	U5

E

Egyptian	*n.*	埃及人（语）	
	adj.	埃及（人）的	U2
element	*n.*	要素；元素；（学科的）基本原则	U3
emission	*n.*	排放，辐射；排放物，散发物（尤指气体）	U3
equilibrium	*n.*	均衡；平静；保持平衡的能力	U4

eventually	*adv.*	终于，最后	U2
excipient	*n.*	赋型剂；药用辅料	U3

F

Father of Botany		植物学之父	U2
flavonoid	*n.*	黄酮类；[有化] 类黄酮	U4
flavor	*vt.*	给……调味；给……增添风趣	U5
fluoride	*n.*	[化] 氟化物	U5

G

galenical	*n.*	草药，未经精炼的药物	U2
	adj.	草本制剂的	U2
glycoside	*n.*	配糖体；配糖类	U4
gravimetric	*adj.*	（测定）重量的，重量分析的	U3

H

has its roots in		根源于	U4
herbal	*adj.*	草药的；草本的	U4
	n.	植物志；草本书	U4
holistic	*adj.*	整体的；全盘的	U4

I

identify	*v.*	鉴定；识别，辨认出；把……看成一样	U3
inactive	*adj.*	不活动的，不活跃的	U5
ingredient	*n.*	（混合物的）组成部分；要素；因素；（烹调的）原料	U3
innovation	*n.*	改革；新观念；新事物；新设施	U1

insight	n.	洞察力，深入了解	U7
inspector	n.	检查员；巡视员	U6
instinct	n.	本能，直觉；天性	U2
	adj.	充满着的	U2
in the light of		根据，按照	U2
investigation	n.	侦查；调查，研究；科学研究；学术研究	U1
invocation	n.	祈求，祈祷	U2
isolated	adj.	偏远的；孤立的，单独的；孤独的；绝缘的	U6

J

jurisdiction	n.	管辖权；管辖范围；权限；司法权	U1

K

Kastle-Meyer	[医]卡-麦二氏试验	U3

L

label	n.	标签；标记；商标	U5
last	vi.	持续	U5
lax	adj.	不严格的，松懈的	U6
list	vt.	列出，列入；把……编列成表；记入名单内	U5
loophole	n.	漏洞；枪眼；换气孔；射弹孔	U6

M

maintain	vt.	保持；保养；坚持；固执己见	U1
manufacturing	n.	制造业，工业	U1
match	vt.	相同；适应；使较量；使等同于	U5

materials	*n.*	素材；材料，原料；布，织物	U1
matrix	*n.*	[数]矩阵；模型；	U3
molecular	*adj.*	分子的，由分子组成的	U7
morphine	*n.*	[药]吗啡	U4

N

numerous	*adj.*	很多的，许多的；数不清的	U3

O

operate	*vt.*	经营；运转；管理	
	vi.	开刀，动手术	U1
opium	*n.*	鸦片；麻醉剂	U4
	adj.	鸦片的	

P

paracetamol	*n.*	对乙酰氨基酚；氨基酚	U3
perusal	*n.*	熟读；精读	U6
pharmaceutical	*adj.*	制药（学）的	U6
pharmacy	*n.*	药房；配药学，药剂学	U2
pill	*n.*	药丸；弹丸	U5
pin	*vt.*	钉住；压住；将……用针别住	U6
	n.	大头针，别针；栓；琐碎物	U6
play a significant role in		在……发挥重要作用	U1
poppy	*n.*	罂粟花；罂粟属植物；深红色	U4
	adj.	罂粟科的	
preclinical	*adj.*	临床前的，潜伏期的；临床使用前的	U7
pregnant	*adj.*	怀孕的；孕育着	U5

prescription	n.	[医]药方，处方；处方药	U5
preservatives	n.	防腐剂；预防法；防护层	U5
primarily	adv.	首先；首要地，主要地；根本上	U3
prior to		在……之前	U3
procedure	n.	程序，手续；工序，步骤	U3
promulgate	vt.	公布；传播；发表	U2
public	adj.	公众的，公共的；政府的	U1
	n.	知名；大众；社会；公共场所	U1

Q

quantitative	adj.	定量的；数量（上）的	U3

R

rather than		而不是；宁可……也不愿	U4
raw	adj.	生的，未加工的；无经验的	U3
registration	n.	登记；注册；挂号	U6
regulation	n.	规则；法规；规章；管制	U5
release	vt.	释放；放开；发布；发行	U3
	n.	释放，排放，解除	U3
responsible	adj.	负有责任的；尽责的；承担责任；懂道理的	U1
restore	vt.	恢复；修复；归还	U6
revered	adj.	可敬的，尊敬的	U2

S

safety	n.	安全；安全性；安全处所；中卫	U1
sample	n.	样品；标本；榜样	U3
	vt.	取……的样品，抽样调查	U3

saponin	n.	肥皂精；[生化] 皂素	U4
self-discipline	n.	自律；自我修养	U6
side effects		副作用；毒副作用；不良作用	U5
significant	adj.	有意义的；有重大意义的；值得注意的	
	n.	有意义的事物；象征，标志	U1
since then		从那时起	U4
solution	n.	解决；溶解；溶液；答案	U3
spectrum	n.	光谱；波谱；范围；系列	U3
spring from		起源于，来自，发源（于）……	U2
stem from		起源于	U2
sterol	n.	[有化] 甾醇；[有化] 固醇	U4
submit	vt.	使服从；主张；呈递；提交	U6
substance	n.	物质，材料；实质，内容；（织品的）质地	U3
supervision	n.	监督，管理	U6
supply	n.	供给物；储备物质；粮食	U1
syrup	n.	糖浆，糖汁；糖浆类药品	U5

T

tablet	n.	碑，匾；药片；便笺簿；小块	U3
teaspoon	n.	茶匙；一茶匙的量	U5
territory	n.	领土，领域；范围；地域；版图	U6
thoroughly	adv.	彻底地，完全地	U6
titration	n.	滴定；滴定法；滴定法测定	U3
titrimetry	n.	滴定分析；滴定测量；滴定分析法	U3
toothpaste	n.	牙膏	U5
toxicity	n.	毒性，毒力	U7
transformation	n.	转化；转变；改造；转型	U3
transparent	adj.	透明的；显然的；坦率的；易懂的	U6
treat	v.	对待；治疗；处理；款待	U5

trial	*n.*	试验；审讯	U7

U

universal	*adj.*	普遍的；通用的；全体的	U6
usage	*n.*	用途	

W

workload	*n.*	工作量	U6

References

[1] 百度文库. 英语后置定语的详细用法 [EB/OL].
https://wenku.baidu.com/view/4eac917402768e9951e738ac.html/2018-06-26.

[2] 百度文库. 过去分词作状语的用法归纳 [EB/OL].
https://wenku.baidu.com/view/843322e2ed630b1c58eeb5a2.html.

[3] 薄冰. 薄冰大学英语语法 [M]. 北京：开明出版社，2017.

[4] *China Daily*. Professional and specialized drug inspectors[EB/OL].
https://www.chinadaily.com.cn/a/201908/05/WS5d476c2aa310cf3e35563d1a.html/2019-08-05.

[5] Christine Ruggeri. Herbal Medicine Benefits [EB/OL].
https://draxe.com/health/herbal-medicine/2017-05-08.

[6] Christopher J Thomsen. "Pharmacy Automation-Practical Technology Solutions for the Pharmacy" (PDF). Business Briefing : US Pharmacy Review 2004. The Thompson Group. Retrieved 5 March 2010.

[7] FDA. The Drug Development Process[EB/OL].
https://www.fda.gov/patients/learn-about-drug-and-device-approvals/drug-development-process/2018-01-04.

[8] George A. Bender. A History of Pharmacy in Pictures [EB/OL].
http://www.doc88.com/p-9085228747684.html/2016-10-06.

[9] Globaledgerecruiting. Pharmaceutical Sales Jobs – Jobs in Pharmaceutical Sales[EB/OL].
https://www.globaledgerecruiting.com/specialties/pharmaceutical.

[10] Information Services Office. Drug Safety and Efficacy Conference[EB/OL].
http://www.iso.cuhk.edu.hk/english/publications/newsletter/article.aspx?articleid=57819/2013-11-19.

[11] Life Alert. Over-the-Counter Medicines:What's Right for You?[EB/OL].
http://lifealert.com/health/countermedicines.aspx.

[12] Liz Parks (November/December 2003 issue). "Market Survey of Pharmacy Technology and Automation in Retail and Outpatient Pharmacy" (PDF). Retail Pharmacy Management. The Thomsen group. Retrieved 6 March 2010.

[13] Michaela Bucheler. English for the Pharmaceutical Industry[M]. Oxford: Oxford University Press, 2010.

[14] Steen Hansen, Stig Pedersen-Bjergaard&Knut Rasmussen. Introduction to Pharmaceutical Chemical Analysis[M]. New Jersey:A John Wiley & Sons, Ltd, 2012.

[15] Woodward English. Passive Voice [EB/OL]. https://www.grammar.cl/Notes/Passive_Voice.htm.